The 7-DAY
Superfood
Cleanse

STEPHANIE PEDERSEN

STERLING
New York

TO MY DETOXERS
Every single one of you!
I have enjoyed every 3-Day, 5-Day, 7-Day, 14-Day, 21-Day,
and 30-Day cleanse I have done with you.
You have taught me so, so much! Thank you!
You are the inspiration for this book.
I adore you!

STERLING
New York

An Imprint of Sterling Publishing
1166 Avenue of the Americas
New York, NY 10036

Text © 2015 by Stephanie Pedersen
Photography © 2015 by Sterling Publishing Co., Inc.
Insert photography by Bill Milne

ISBN 978-1-4549-1623-9

Distributed in Canada by Sterling Publishing
c/o Canadian Manda Group, 664 Annette Street
Toronto, Ontario, Canada M6S 2C8
Distributed in the United Kingdom by GMC Distribution Services
Castle Place, 166 High Street, Lewes, East Sussex, England BN7 1XU
Distributed in Australia by Capricorn Link (Australia) Pty. Ltd.
P.O. Box 704, Windsor, NSW 2756, Australia

For information about custom editions, special sales, and premium
and corporate purchases, please contact Sterling Special Sales
at 800-805-5489 or specialsales@sterlingpublishing.com

Manufactured in Canada

2 4 6 8 10 9 7 5 3 1

www.sterlingpublishing.com

CONTENTS

Introduction iv

1 The 7-Day Superfood Cleanse:
What it Is and How it Works 1

2 Setting Goals and Getting into the Zone 10

3 How it All Works 23

4 Green Drinks, Smoothies, and Other Detox Drinks 45

5 Breakfast 69

6 Lunch 76

7 Snacks 98

8 Dinner 115

9 Detox Self-Care 132

10 Coming Off the Detox 147

11 Extending Your Cleanse 152

12 Pop-Up Cleanses 154

13 Troubleshooting 156

14 Detox FAQs 164

Resources 171
Metric Equivalents Charts 175
Acknowledgments 176
Index 178
About the Author 184

INTRODUCTION:
WHY A BOOK ON DETOXING?

CLEANSES ARE HOT RIGHT NOW, AND with good reason: A cleanse gives you a short break from foods that leave you feeling bloated, sluggish, and overweight (and also sap your energy, affect your blood sugar, cause cravings, and make you look older). In return, you slim down—often one or two dress sizes!—lose the puffiness, feel more energetic than ever, experience life without cravings, and look and feel younger than ever. It sounds almost too good to be true, doesn't it? But I assure you that a cleanse can do all of these things and so much more, including clear up your skin, regulate your sleep, help you lose your taste for junk and carb-laden food, and make you more mentally focused than ever.

But not all cleanses are the same. The 7-Day Superfood Cleanse harnesses the power of nature's most nutrient-dense *superfoods* to detox deeply, safely, and quickly in order to help you look and feel at your best!

But first, what is a detox? Detoxes, cleanses, fasts, reboots, resets, and so on are all names for the same thing: a short, drink-based (or drink-and-food-based) diet designed to help you drop bloat and water weight very quickly, shed a few pounds, shrink a dress size or more, ditch certain food cravings, excrete stored toxins (such as parabens, BPA, phthalates, mercury, arsenic, lead, antimony, aluminum, petroleum by-products, pesticides, and other additives—all of which have been found in food, supplements, cleaning supplies, shampoos, lotions, deodorants, makeup, and so on), clear up your skin, cut through brain fog, and become reacclimatized to healthy eating.

Detoxes can last anywhere from a long weekend to several months and may or may not include a few whole foods. Some programs are designed to speed the loss of water weight and toxins through lymph drainage massage, sweating, detox breathing, body brushing, body wraps, and even more controversial practices such as enemas and colonics.

Cleanses are all the rage right now because they work. They really do.

BENEFITS OF CLEANSING

Thanks to the fast release of water weight, you can easily lose five pounds in three days, and double that in a week. The quality of your skin noticeably improves, creating the "detox glow" that people talk about. Cravings for sweets and carbohydrates disappear, thanks to all the vegetable juices that are consumed while cleansing. At the same time, sleep improves, mood improves, and focus and mental acuity improve.

As these many changes take place, you begin to feel and look healthier while enjoying a renewed sense of self-esteem. Suddenly, overeating and eating junk food isn't appealing. You now want to continue to eat healthfully and take care of yourself. And you really do feel as if your eating habits and overall health have been reset.

These are some of the many benefits you'll enjoy from the 7-Day Superfood Cleanse:

- Fast, significant weight loss, due to the quick release of water weight
- Dropping one or more dress sizes
- Losing belly bloat
- Getting rid of face and neck puffiness, including under-eye bags, puffy eyes, double chin, and jowls
- Acquiring the "detox glow" from an increase in antioxidant intake
- Clearer, brighter eyes
- Getting rid of the strong sugar, carbohydrate, and caffeine cravings that many of us grapple with
- Discovering a healthier way to eat over the long term
- Feeling cleaner and lighter
- Feeling less irritable and enjoying more stable moods
- Increased mental acuity and focus
- More physical and mental stamina and energy
- Improved sleep

- Heightened intuition and creativity
- More efficient digestion
- A decrease in environmental allergies and food intolerances
- Reduction in toxic load from chemicals in plastics, cleaning products, cosmetics, and so on
- Faster healing from injuries
- Improved immune system function
- A new way of seeing and using food

THE WHY AND HOW OF CLEANSING

The main purpose of a cleanse is to use (and, ideally, to enjoy) special "detoxifying" foods that encourage your body to quickly and aggressively excrete water weight, which is where your body typically stores the majority of the toxins ingested from junk food and beverages, polluted air and water, and chemicals in automobile and housecleaning products, as well as cosmetics and self-care products, such as deodorants, shampoos, and many other body "cleansers."

You can speed up a detox even more by consuming cleansing ingredients in liquid form—juice or smoothies, for example. Liquid detoxes give your digestive system a break, allowing your body to use the energy from these beverages as fuel to help the cleansing process go even deeper, pushing out additional, deeply stored toxins and water weight. As toxins leave the body, and as your body is flooded with high levels of antioxidants, the functioning of your nervous, immune, and digestive systems dramatically improves. In short, you look—and feel—amazing.

WHAT MAKES THIS CLEANSE DIFFERENT?

Despite all of the obvious advantages of cleansing, detoxing can be challenging. Subsisting on a narrow diet of just a few sanctioned foods can rob your body of much-needed nutrients, causing you to feel a lot worse than you should. This is my biggest pet peeve about other detoxes! No one should have to go through a cleanse without the support of health-boosting, nutritional foods. That's the reason I insist that the people I work with in my private practice use a carefully chosen array of powerful, nutrient-dense superfoods. I don't think it makes any sense at all to feel bad or compromise your health in order to look better, which is why I feel so passionate about sharing what I've discovered—and what has proven to be so successful about my detoxing methods—with you in *The 7-Day Superfood Cleanse*.

THE SUPERFOOD CONNECTION

In the pages that follow, I'll explain what superfoods are and what makes them so super, not only for your health in general, but also for cleansing in particular. You'll find dozens of delicious recipes and menus that feature this special group of foods and discover how integrating them into your detox regimen will help you stay on track and achieve your weight loss and health goals—without feeling grumpy, tired, hungry, or anxious. With an assortment of blender drinks, juices, teas, and other beverages for detox breakfasts, such as my signature green drink (which you can customize, depending upon the ingredients that suit you), and heartier fare, such as Braised Coconut Spinach and Chickpeas with Lemon and Quinoa Superfood Salad for lunch and dinner—not to mention Chia Pudding or Kale Chips whenever you feel the need for a snack—the 7-Day Superfood Cleanse not only keeps you healthy while you detox, but it also shows you how to safely come off the cleanse and stay away from unhealthy eating habits. There's even a section on detox self-care products to help support your cleanse from the outside in, by preventing the reintroduction of the very same toxins you are working so hard to elimininate.

THE ADVANTAGES OF A SHORT CLEANSE

Then there's the emotional piece of cleansing that no one wants to talk about but happens to be the biggest reason why people quit when they're halfway through: Giving up your favorite foods can be tough, and relying on drinks (when you love to crunch and chew!) can be a real challenge. Who wants to eat clean and green (and only fluids!) when everyone around you is enjoying the foods you love to eat?

That's why shorter detoxes, such as the 7-Day Superfood Cleanse, have the highest success rates. As more research is done on fasting, a growing number of physicians are touting the benefits of occasional short fasts. For instance, Dr. Andrew Weil and Dr. Mehmet Oz—both of whom are also health authors and healthy-eating advocates—advocate periodic one- to three-day fasts as an easy way stay healthy and keep clean and fit.

"Quick cleanses" are also healthier options for most people, since they don't require the close (and sometimes constant) medical supervision of longer, more extreme detoxing. However, if you do want a longer period in which to detox, and if your healthcare provider feels you're up to it, the 7-Day Superfood Cleanse gives you the option to safely extend cleansing to 10 or more days, and gives you other choices as well, such as using occasional 1-day fasts to help jump-start weight-loss, kick carb cravings, or help treat a health condition.

ARE YOU READY?

So, are you ready to dive in and change your health—and yes, even your life? I am so excited about inviting you to join me on the 7-Day Superfood Cleanse! You're going to discover how delicious, nutrient-dense foods will help you harness the power of detoxing to lose weight, maintain weight loss, and feel great. I'm equally passionate about making the process as enjoyable as possible, because if you want to get through a detox and glean all of the benefits, you need to have some fun!

I look forward to detoxing with you.

Enjoy!

Stephanie Pedersen, MS, CHHC
www.StephaniePedersen.com

THE 7-DAY SUPERFOOD CLEANSE: WHAT IT IS AND HOW IT WORKS

THANK YOU FOR BECOMING A DETOXER! That's what I call anyone who goes through one of my cleanse programs. You are going to have a great time cleaning up your health and losing weight. You'll feel fantastic and look fantastic. You'll also find new levels of energy, focus, creativity, and intuition that you may not have dreamed possible.

You've probably noticed that there are many detoxes available right now, from prepackaged 3-day juice-only regimens (typically created by bottled juice companies) to 21-day water-lemon-honey-and-cayenne fasts (think Master Cleanse) to whole food "reboots" designed to jump-start your return to healthy eating. You'll find simple whole food reboots popular with wellness and health coaches, liquid fasts administered by nutritionists and naturopaths, and raw food detoxes created by local raw food restaurants. There are shake-based 5-day programs (typically ped-aled by multilevel marketing vitamin sellers) and green powder drink kits. There are herbal liver cleanses, sugar blues boot camp fasts, and even big-gun medical detoxes designed to rid the body of heavy metals and toxins, such as the parabens found in cosmetics and cleaning products, and BPA in plastic water bottles. And there are plenty of other cleanses that you may not have heard of.

In short, there's a whole lot of cleansing going on! Most of these programs are done by individuals on their own, people who love the idea of losing weight, bloat, and cravings (as well as improving their energy, sleep, focus, and the quality of their skin) in a short amount of time.

It's a terrific concept: You spend a short amount of time going deep, clearing out the foods and toxins that leave you feeling puffy, bloated, and sluggish and affect the quality of your skin and hair, too. In return, you lose a few (or more than a few) pounds, ditch the cravings that make healthy eating difficult, enjoy a brighter and firmer complexion, drop a dress size or two, and feel vibrant and full of energy.

All of this is possible with a cleanse. But—there's always a *but*, right?—it's important to detox in a way that doesn't leave you feeling spent, irritable, jittery, cold, weak, and hungry. And you don't want a cleanse to have negative effects on your skin, hair, sleep, or energy, either. What many people don't realize, however, is that any time you reduce your food intake, you also run the risk of running low on the nutrients that help you look and feel your best. In my opinion, this completely negates the point of detoxing for health!

SUPERFOODS, WEIGHT LOSS, AND YOUR HEALTH

That's why I created the 7-Day Superfood Cleanse: I want my clients to be deeply supported by nutrient-dense ingredients while they cleanse their bodies of trapped water weight, questionable food ingredients, and toxins. At the same time, I want them to experience a physical and emotional break from the addictive, acid-forming foods that set them up for uncontrollable cravings, unstable blood sugar, sleep disturbances, water retention, low-grade aches and pains, fatigue, mental slowness, mood swings, and a generally un-vibrant demeanor.

Superfoods, also known as power foods or functional foods, are at the foundation of the 7-Day Superfood Cleanse. These deeply nourishing plant foods (such as tea, nuts, seeds, whole grains, and legumes) contain thousands of phytonutrients (also known as phytochemicals) and are popular among health professionals and nutritionists because they help prevent disease and keep our bodies working properly.

Thus, the secret of the 7-Day Superfood Cleanse is twofold: It removes foods that detract from your looks and overall health, while supplying the nutritional powerhouses that supercharge healing, weight loss, energy levels, and your natural good looks. At the same time, you detox faster, deeper, easier, and more comfortably. How's that for a proposition?

THE POWER OF SUPERFOODS

I know firsthand how powerful superfoods are. I have used them to help heal my oldest son's eczema and heavy metal poisoning; I have used them to make learning easier for my second son, who has dyslexia; and I have used them to keep my youngest son cold-free when everyone in his class comes down with a virus. My husband uses superfoods to keep his blood pressure low and cardiovascular system strong. I use them to help my skin look great, keep my energy levels high, and treat unexpected bloat—and of course they've played starring roles in my own quarterly personal detoxes.

Here are some of my favorite superfood ingredients and how I like to use them.

- AVOCADO: Avocados are not only delicious, but also rich in glutathione, a nutrient that helps inactivate toxins by forcing toxins from the body through the kidneys and urine. Avocados also are rich in carotenoids to support a healthy immune sytem (which also helps remove toxins from the body) and anti-inflammatory fatty acids to help with cardiovascular health. Avocados have been shown in research studies to help promote blood sugar regulation—necessary to quell the carb and sugar cravings that take out many a detoxer. In the 7-Day Superfood Cleanse, you'll find avocados in your morning green drink, as well as in salads, quinoa, and bean bowls, and as guacamole and dip.
- CHIA: I fell in love with chia when I co-wrote *Chia: The Complete Guide to the World's Ultimate Superfood* (Sterling) with Dr. Wayne Coates. A tiny black seed, chia packs a nutritional wallop, thanks to protein, omega-3 fatty acids, soluble fiber, phytonutrients, and a host of vitamins and minerals. Extreme athletes use chia for energy, hydration, and muscle repair. I use it to help my skin glow and stay healthy, to increase mental acuity and focus, and to help ward off carb cravings—all of which are going to help you, beautiful detoxer, stay on the program, look great, and feel fantastic. I love using chia in Chia Fresca (a refreshing snack drink) and Chia Pudding, found in the snack chapter. You'll also have the option to take advantage of chia's energizing qualities by adding it to your morning green drink.

- COCONUT: I have always loved coconut. Not only is the taste divine, it also comes in so many enjoyable-to-use forms, from water to oil, meat to flour. My favorites are coconut milk (which I use in place of dairy in recipes) and oil (great for sautéing and as a beauty aid). I aim for at least one serving of some form of coconut every day, which gives me a daily supply of medium-chain fatty acids for heart and brain health and a strong immune system. You'll find some form of coconut in almost every recipe in the 7-Day Superfood Cleanse, from drinks to soups to snacks. I love its strong antimicrobial activity, which helps the body clear viruses, bacteria, and fungi. The fiber in coconut flour and coconut meat is terrific at lowering food's glycemic index and filling you up, meaning you are full with less food! And the medium-chain fatty acids help the heart, are anti-inflammatories, and are said to help with brain health.
- CRANBERRY: Some people have a sweet tooth. Me? I have a sour tooth, which is why I adore cranberries. I juice them raw—daily if I am experiencing breakouts or another complexion glitch. The berry contains large amounts of anthocyanins, an antioxidant with strong anti-inflammatory power which also helps ward off urinary tract infections, boosts cardiovascular health, and aids in preventing cancer and liver disease. You'll find them in the 7-Day Superfood Cleanse signature *Winter Pink Drink* (pages 59–60).
- KALE (AND OTHER GREENS): I have always loved kale, so much so that I wrote *Kale: A Complete Guide to the World's Most Powerful Superfood* (Sterling). I love the taste of kale but it's the nutrients that keep me coming back for more: omega-3 fatty acids, fiber, chlorophyll, minerals, antioxidant flavonoids, protein, vitamins K, A, and C. I call for kale as an optional green drink ingredient, as a snack food (check out the kale chips recipes on pages 107–108), and in salad.
- PEPITAS: These green, hulless pumpkin seeds are one of my favorite foods. I toss them into jarred salsa, salads, sandwich fillings, and granola; sprinkle them over soup; use them as a garnish for Mexican food; and eat them dry-popped and seasoned with tamari. Every time I enjoy them, I am getting large amounts of manganese, zinc,

phosphorus, vitamin E, fiber, and protein, not to mention phytonutrients, all of which help prevent cancer, cardiovascular disease, and diabetes. They are used to add high-quality vegan protein and fiber to salads and grain and bean dishes in the 7-Day Superfood Cleanse.

• POMEGRANATE: Pomegranates have always been in my life. They grew wild on my maternal grandparents' property, so my grandmother would send jars of homemade pomegranate jelly to us. When my family moved to the United States from Australia, we, too, set up house on land with two wild pomegranate trees. There were few things I liked more as a kid than eating pomegranate seeds. Little did I know then that I was doing my immune system a favor, thanks to the seeds' high vitamin C, K, and B_5 content, as well as fiber and anti-inflammatory phytonutrients. I use them in several 7-Day Superfood Cleanse drinks and salads because they have three times as many antioxidants as red wine and green tea and contain three types of polyphenols—tannins, athocyanins, and ellagic acid—all of which support the body's ability to flush toxins.

• QUINOA: The darling of the healthy-eating set, quinoa is a small seed that is used as a culinary grain. In my world, it is a stand-in for rice, but with a much higher protein content that makes it a perfect alternative to animal protein during a detox (which is always vegan). Quinoa also boasts fiber, manganese, magnesium, omega-3 fatty acids, and antioxidant flavonoids and helps alkalize the body so it can secrete toxins more efficiently. You'll find it in a variety of pilaf, grain bowl, and salad recipes here in the 7-Day Superfood Cleanse.

• WALNUTS: Crunchy, slightly bitter, and meaty, walnuts are my go-to ingredient when I want a toothsome hit of protein for a salad or as a garnish. Just a quarter cup with give you around 94 percent of your body's daily requirement for omega-3 fatty acids. They also offer manganese, molybdenum, vitamin E, protein, and fiber to benefit every body system. And because they are high in the toxin-flushing ingredient glutathione, they are used in many of the salad, grain, and bean recipes within the 7-Day Superfood Cleanse. You'll also see them listed as an optional ingredient in your morning green drink!

HOW DO YOU KNOW
IF A DETOX IS FOR YOU?

1. Have you gained weight recently that you have been unable to lose?

2. Are you puffy, bloated, or soft anywhere in your body or face?

3. Do you need caffeine to start your day? Or, do you rely on caffeine in the middle of the day to maintain your productivity?

4. Do you crave sweets? Crunchy, salty foods? Creamy foods? Alcohol? Tobacco? Caffeine? Do you consider yourself addicted to chips, cookies, chocolate, ice cream, pastries, bread, coffee, wine, or other health-sapping foods?

5. Do you drag through your days?

6. Has your mojo disappeared? (Or, worse, have you never had any mojo?)

7. Are you living without passion? Without spark? Without enthusiasm?

8. Do you have trouble winding down at night in order to get to bed?

9. Do you suffer from brain fog? Do you wish you were sharper? More creative? More intuitive?

10. Is it hard to get motivated to work? Do you have trouble sustaining focus?

11. Have you had candida or a series of viruses or fungal or bacterial infections in the last year or more that you don't feel fully recovered from?

If you answered *yes* to two or more of these questions, detoxing could be just what you need to feel and look lighter, clearer, and more glowing and achieve a massive increase in energy, intuition, creativity, and motivation. A short detox is a powerful way to jump-start a committed weight loss program, improve the quality of your skin, improve digestive issues, discover food intolerances, improve mental acuity, feel lighter and more energetic, as well as eliminate addictions to sugary or carb-laden food, caffeine, alcohol, and other health-sapping foods.

If you have an eating or exercise disorder, a distorted body image, HIV, diabetes, or hypoglycemia, or if you are pregnant, an emotional eater, or recovering from a serious illness, you should not undertake a cleanse without the explicit permission and supervision of your health care provider.

ARE YOU READY TO GET STARTED? LET'S GO!

You've read about what a cleanse is and what the 7-Day Superfood Cleanse contains. But what, exactly, will you be doing for the next 7 days?

Good question!

You will be eating whole, cleansing plant foods—either in some of the recipes provided here or in pre-made items— and drinking beautiful, energizing green and pink drinks (homemade or store-bought), as well as enjoying various teas. Not just any foods will, do, however. I've chosen combinations that maximize nutrients and detoxification, while simultaneously helping the body squelch cravings and boost the energy levels you'll need to get through your days. I know how important that last detail is: No one has 7 days to spend, sequestered, "doing a detox." It's important to be able to go about your everyday life feeling as good as possible. And you will!

Let me give you a little look at what you'll be up to during the 7-Day Superfood Cleanse. Each day you'll be starting with a specially made green drink, made fresh just for you, using ingredients that suit you best. (You can purchase your green drinks if you'd prefer.) If you look at chapters 4 and 5, you'll see that I give you instructions on how to customize your green drink to suit your individual needs. Can't have kale? Use romaine. Cucumbers make you burp? Leave them out. Hate the taste of lemon? Use lime. This green drink is the cornerstone of my program and ensures that you start the day energized, alkalized (more soon on why this is important), and craving-free.

To help you lose weight, feel light and healthy, and be your most energetic, you'll be following one of two special plans.

THE EVERYDAY CLEANSE PLAN

The Everyday Cleanse Plan features high-protein lunches, optional twice-daily snacks, and a light dinner (to best facilitate weight loss). Most of the calories you'll take in will be consumed midday to boost weight loss and get rid of trapped water.

You'll find recipes for lunch dishes in chapter 6. All the recipes are easy to make ahead, tote to work, or enjoy at home. You'll dig in to delicious foods like *Coconut Quinoa* (page 90) with *Braised Coconut Spinach and Chickpeas with Lemon* (page 93)—or your own signature creation, using the *Grain or Bean Salad Blueprint* (page 80). The section on toxin-free food containers is a must-read, and you'll find other important information and tips about weight loss and detoxing—the reasons why eating at your desk is not a good idea, for example. If you're a takeout fan, you'll find a comprehensive list of great, easy buy-and-go options—perfect for those of you who don't enjoy cooking (or don't have the time to cook).

Snacks are an important part of many of our days, and while I do not allow chips, cookies, or the like, chapter 7 features some delicious options for snacking, including *Avocado-Coconut Dip* (page 113), several types of hummus, kale chips, *Chia Pudding* (page 101), and my favorite, *Chia Fresca* (page 100).

Dinners on the cleanse are light and easily digested so your body can do the heavy lifting of detoxing while you sleep. In chapter 8 you'll find a wide array of soups, from *Superfood Beet Soup* (page 119) to *Spicy Pumpkin Coconut Bisque* (page 118), as well as dinner salads (my favorite is the *Chopped Avocado Coconut Salad*, page 124) and scrumptious healthy salad dressings. There's a lot of information about late-night snacking in this chapter, as well as a phenomenon known as "coming down off the day," a time when many people are prone to stress eating.

THE QUICK CLEANSE PLAN

The Quick Cleanse Plan is designed for detoxers who want to push the envelope a bit. It is a modified liquid fast using green drinks and other superfood-filled beverages (and solid foods at lunch) to help release double the amount of trapped water and toxins that are lost with the Everyday Cleanse Plan and further accelerate weight loss. It's a restrictive menu that is not meant to be used for more than two days (and not consecutive days, at that, which is why I ask you to try it only on days 4 and 6). It is the menu I use whenever I wake up feeling puffy and need to fit into a special dress that night or the next day.

You'll find all the nuts and bolts of the 7-Day Superfood Cleanse program in chapter 3. I can't wait for you to have a look!

But for now, I invite you to turn to chapter 2, where I talk about something essential to a successful cleanse: getting into the zone! This is where I'll show you how to prepare your mind, body, and kitchen so that you can dive headfirst into success. Look for a goal sheet, on which I ask you to actually write down your goals for the detox as a powerful way to begin your 7-Day Superfood Cleanse.

Have fun!

SETTING GOALS
AND GETTING INTO THE ZONE

Y AY! YOU ARE JUMPING INTO the 7-Day Superfood Cleanse! You are going to have a great time cleaning up your health and losing weight. You'll feel fantastic and look fantastic. You'll also find new levels of energy, focus, creativity, and intuition that you may not have thought possible.

Let me start by asking you a couple of questions, the same ones I ask every single person in my detox groups:

1. What is your goal? What do you want to get from the 7-Day Superfood Cleanse?
2. What are you willing to do in order to achieve your goal?

Maybe you want to lose weight. Or finally get rid of your sugar cravings. Or learn to live without coffee. Or explore a plant-based diet. Maybe you want to stop feeling bloated, get more energy, clean up your skin, become more intuitive, sharpen your mental faculties, or strengthen your immune system. Cleansing your body of toxins and stored chemicals is a great way to start achieving any of those goals. The beauty of the 7-Day Superfood Cleanse is that it will improve your health over the long term—no matter what your immediate goals may be.

Use the questions in the box to create your own goal sheet. Place your goal sheet somewhere where you can see it often. Committing to a goal in writing is powerful: It not only acts as a reminder of what you want to achieve (which is important when your attention starts to wane and it becomes all too easy to lose sight of the prize), but also motivates you, by giving you a result to work toward. This is truly important. Of all my clients, the ones who publicly state their intentions for change are the ones who are most likely to successfully achieve their goals.

MY 7-DAY SUPERFOOD CLEANSE HEALTH GOALS

I want to look and feel healthy this year. So, what will I do differently right now to finally look and feel healthy this year?

HEALTH GOAL 1:

(SAMPLE)

I want to *lose 5 pounds*.

Because I am *tired of not fitting into my jeans*.

The action steps I will take to achieve this goal are:

1. *Participate in the 7-Day Superfood Cleanse with Stephanie*
2. *Exercise for 30 minutes each day*
3. *Get 8 hours of sleep each evening*
4. *Stop eating after 7:30 each evening*

HEALTH GOAL 2:

I want to _____

Because I am _____

The action steps I will take to achieve this goal are:

1.
2.
3.
4.

GETTING READY TO CLEANSE

Did you complete your goal sheet? Fantastic! Now on to the next order of business: getting yourself in the zone. This is an interesting place to be, a place ruled by mindset and physical preparation. Some people do not need this—they can dive into new things easily, with no particular need to become acclimated. Most of us, however, need to consider the possibilities and decide the best way to make something happen before plunging in. If that is you, then this chapter is a must-read.

Here I'll give you a few pre-detox assignments, which you can do the day or week or even month beforehand—starting right this moment, if you'd like—to ensure that your experience with the 7-Day Superfood Cleanse is as smooth, easy, and enjoyable as possible.

INCREASE YOUR WATER INTAKE

Your first assignment is a critical one, because your body needs water to flush toxins, help eliminate stored fat, and be well lubricated. Ready?

Sip water throughout the day. Feel free to add lemon or lime juice, apple cider vinegar, or cucumber slices to your glass of water. I suggest that you keep water with you at all times, just so you have it handy. At this point, I am not going to tell you to drink a specific amount; just be mindful of drinking water.

Starting tomorrow morning, before you put anything else in your body, drink a large glass of lukewarm water (not cold!) with a squirt (about 1 teaspoon) of lemon or lime juice or a splash of apple cider vinegar.

Do you dislike drinking water? If so, why? What can you do to make water drinking more pleasant for you?

ELIMINATE COFFEE

Are you addicted to coffee? How do you feel about giving it up during a detox?

For the javaheads among you, have you gone coffee-free yet? If not, now is the time to dive in and take a bold step!

Eliminating coffee right now will make your cleanse so much more comfortable. Yes, you have to give up your coffee—or most of

WHY DRINK APPLE CIDER VINEGAR?

Apple cider vinegar is made from crushed and fermented apples (in the old days, it was made from apples that were too old and mushy to be eaten whole or used for baking). As the juice is released during fermentation, natural bacteria are introduced from the environment, which, in turn, lead to the formation of acetic acid, a powerful antimicrobial agent and disinfectant that helps rid the body—both topically and internally—of pathogens that can make you sick. This is why apple cider vinegar has been used for cleaning wounds (Hippocrates wrote about this!), fighting internal infections and viruses, and preserving foods in the form of pickles. (Try using apple cider vinegar to clean cutting boards and countertops—it's very effective!) Some studies on animals have found that apple cider vinegar helps treat type 2 diabetes, shrink cancerous tumors, reduce blood pressure, strengthen the immune system, help flush stored heavy metals from the body, and squash sugar and carbohydrate cravings.

While I am not a research scientist, I am a big fan of apple cider vinegar. Here's why: I have noticed that when my clients and I ingest apple cider vinegar—as well as many other foods in the 7-Day Superfood Cleanse—we are less likely to be hungry for sugary, carb-laden foods, such as muffins, pastries, double Frappuccino lattes, and so on, which adversely affect our blood sugar and do nothing to support our health. Consuming these foods sends us into a cycle of giving in to what we crave and, subsequently, craving more. In short, apple cider vinegar stops this cycle and makes it easier to stick to a plan of healthful eating. For anyone on a cleanse this is great news: Here's a food that actually helps you feel indifferent to the charms of an apple turnover! I ask all detoxers to start their day with a splash of apple cider vinegar—or a splash of lemon or lime juice, which has a similar effect—in order to get immediate protection from cravings. That's what I call setting yourself up for success!

it, anyway! That's the bad news. The good news is you can replace it with black tea (Irish breakfast, Earl Grey, chai-flavored, and so on, but without dairy milk, of course; I explain why on page 65).

If you're drinking more than two cups of coffee a day, I want you to decrease your consumption to one small cup. Yes, I am trusting you here. I know you know what a small cup is. If you want more caffeine during the day, you can go with black tea (a splash of almond or coconut milk with it is fine) or green tea.

Why is coffee a no-no for detoxing? It plays tricks with your blood sugar, causing powerful simple-carb cravings in a way that tea doesn't. Coffee consumption also forces the adrenal glands to release cortisol into the body, which causes an unnatural and unnecessary fight-or-flight response. When this happens your body is focused on fleeing from a perceived threat (emphasis on the word perceived); too much coffee, sugar, or other stimulants can mimic the very real and urgent reactions your body would actually go through if you were running away from a real threat, such as a saber-toothed tiger. In this scenario (real or perceived) your energy is diverted from regeneration, healing, digesting, flushing toxins, and eliminating waste. With time, your body's systems don't operate as efficiently as they should, and you may notice that you feel fatigued, bloated, moody, unfocused, and wan; be plagued with skin conditions and carb cravings, and fall prey to every virus that comes your way. In other words, a body full of cortisol is not a body that can flush toxins! Last, coffee creates big-time body bloat—especially if you're a woman. Go a few days without coffee, and you'll see how much more svelte you feel and how much better your face looks.

If you find yourself craving coffee or experiencing a withdrawal headache, an extra green drink (page 45) or water with lemon juice or apple cider vinegar can really help!

Be prepared for headaches if coffee has been an important part of your life. These headaches occur as your body adjusts to life without an addictive substance (you may experience headaches when you cut out sugar, alcohol, wheat, and chemical ingredients, as well). You'll notice that withdrawal headaches last for about two days—and you'll soon discover that green drinks can help squash them.

Be prepared to make the switch to a brewed cup of tea (go ahead and get it supersized, if you must) when you find yourself in settings where you may have once habitually grabbed coffee, such as in Starbucks. Don't grab a chai latte, though: The sugar and artificial flavorings will only interfere with your detox and cause cravings, which you'll have to deal with later.

REDUCE OR ELIMINATE ANIMAL FOODS

When we detox, we remove animal-sourced foods from our diets, that is, anything an animal had to die for in order to provide, or anything that comes from a living animal, such as eggs and dairy. (Those of you who have done cleanses before have probably noticed that they are always vegan.)

In my experience with clients on detox programs, I've noticed that there is often resistance to the elimination of meat, so let me spend a little time to give you my take on animal foods. I have no problem with most animal-sourced foods. They provide high doses of protein and, in many cases, healthy fats. For some people who do not metabolize protein efficiently, animal products supply protein and B vitamins that are more easily digestible than those in plant foods.

Because I get many questions from my clients about my own personal diet, I am happy to share that, too. I like to have a splash of dairy milk in my tea and—while I eat a primarily vegan diet—I usually have a serving of some type of meat, poultry, or seafood at least once or twice a week. If I find myself in a restaurant and see mussels on the menu, for example, I will almost always try to convince someone to split an order of them with me.

But—and yes, there's a *but*—animal products *do* create an acidic environment in the body that strongly hampers detoxification. My carnivorous clients and those on the Paleo or South Beach diet hate hearing this, but I have to be honest with you: If you want to detox, you need to allow yourself a short break from animal products. It's as simple

A WORD ABOUT DAIRY AND WEIGHT LOSS

One of the questions I get from clients, especially from women, in every one of my programs is, "Why don't you like yogurt or cottage cheese as a snack or meal food?" (For some reason this isn't a big deal for my male clients.) My answer is that there are so many foods that I truly love—from lemon curd to Campari—but I know they aren't going to help me maintain my health if I eat them on a daily basis. But, boy, sitting with a spoon and a cup of lemon curd is heaven, and in that moment I feel pretty good! I can even trick myself into believing that the high vitamin C content and the protein are giving me some benefit. Which they are—but at the price of health-sapping sugar. It's better for me to get my vitamin C and my protein another way. Right?

But this conversation isn't really about lemon curd or Campari; it's about dairy.

Why don't I love dairy for people who are trying to lose weight or maintain a weight loss? There're a couple of reasons. For one, I've found that women, in particular, don't lose weight or maintain weight loss as easily as men when they eat dairy on a daily basis. A splash of milk in your morning coffee or tea and an occasional cream soup or slice of cheesecake in a restaurant is a lot different than eating cheese or a cup of yogurt every single day, even if they're low-fat.

When I was studying nutrition, one of my instructors mentioned that if a woman keeps yo-yoing or has very slow weight loss without an underlying medical condition, despite all of her attempts to lose weight, there are typically a handful of reasons why. The consumption of dairy was given as one of the top reasons. He also mentioned that people (especially women) can get very emotional if you ask them to remove dairy from their diet. In my experience, I've found this to be true.

There are not a lot of scientific studies in Western medicine to back up my instructor's theory about dairy as an obstacle to weight loss, particularly among women. The dairy industries in the United States, Canada, and Australia are incredibly powerful, and the money spent on pushing various dairy products as "health food" is huge. In traditional Chinese medicine, however, there is plenty of conversation about how dairy creates mucus, inflammation, and acidity, which make the body (including metabolism) run less efficiently, and how it can often set people up for later cravings and affect how the skin looks. I have found that this is true of myself and my family and clients. The moment you finally take a break from dairy is when you'll see bigger weight loss.

There is also an emotional impact (once again, particularly among women) when dairy is taken out of the dietary equation. When I first started practicing, Greek yogurt hadn't become the popular food that it is now, and when I would ask women to take a break from cottage cheese or mozzarella string cheese or yogurt, they would get upset, but not too upset. But now . . . wow, there is something powerful about Greek yogurt! In every program I run, and with each of my private clients, I get emails, calls, and postings from women who are genuinely upset at the thought of doing without Greek yogurt. For some reason, it's always Greek yogurt—probably because it creates a nice sedating cocoon with all that creamy thickness!

So, back to you. How often are you eating dairy? And what do you notice a half hour or an hour or 90 minutes after you eat it? Are you energetic and ready to go? Peppy and mentally alert and focused? Or are you still kind of sedated and comforted? Do you get upset or anxious if you can't have it? Over the course of the 7-Day Superfood Cleanse, there'll be a lot of conversation about our relationship with food.

While you're with me now, however, I'm going to ask you to watch the dairy.

as that and shouldn't be a big deal, since, after all, the 7-Day Superfood Cleanse is only 7 days long! I urge you to give it a try.

To make your cleanse more comfortable, try cutting down on animal products right now, while eating more plant-based protein foods, such as beans, peas, legumes, quinoa, chia, nuts, and seeds, as well as dark leafy greens (yes, they contain protein!). You'll find that plant protein doesn't give you the heavy, stuffed feeling that so many people associate with having "eaten their fill." Get used to the lighter feeling of plant protein now and you'll feel much more comfortable when you get around to doing the 7-Day Superfood Cleanse.

REDUCE OR ELIMINATE FOODS CONTAINING GLUTEN

Gluten, a protein that is present in wheat, is widely used in commercial and homemade baked goods. Gluten is also found in semolina, durum, barley, rye, spelt, and triticale (a cross between wheat and rye). Gluten helps dough to rise and lends shape and a chewy texture to baked goods. It also gives us that mellow, sedative cocoon we all know so well.

When my oldest son was an infant, he was diagnosed with heavy metal toxicity. One of the things our nutritionist asked us to do to help him heal was to remove all gluten from his diet. There were several reasons for this, principally that gluten hampers the body's ability to release stored toxins. Perhaps you've noticed that you feel bloated and puffy after eating gluten-heavy foods. Gluten encourages the body to hold on to the water weight that makes us feel "squishy." It also acidifies the body, further slowing down important body functions, such as metabolism. Gluten also creates a seductive, foggy, numbing state that makes it a favorite comfort food ingredient for stressed or overstretched individuals. Unfortunately, gluten is highly addictive, and the more you eat, the more you want, setting yourself up for a ferocious cycle of craving-gluten-craving-gluten—not something you want to be dealing with while on a cleanse! Your energy is better spent on getting thin and healthy!

REDUCE OR ELIMINATE SOY

I am not a fan of soy. There, I've said it. My vegan clients hate hearing that I do not love meat analogs (you know the ones: soy posing as chorizo), but my job is to help you make the best possible choices for your health—and that often means making informed choices. I like soy even less as an ingredient in a detox program. That's why those prepackaged soy-based shake regimens leave me rolling my eyes (which I know is rude, so I only do it where no one can see me).

The purpose of a detox is to spend a period of time cleaning up your diet and eating foods that promote the flushing of stored toxins and water, and help you to actually crave health-supportive foods instead of health-sapping foods. Soy, however, is higher in phytoestrogens than just about any other food source and has been implicated in a range of hormone-based cancers in both men and women, including breast, endometrial, cervical, ovarian, and prostate cancer. Soy is highly goitrogenic, which means it suppresses thyroid function. When your thyroid doesn't work well, you gain weight, feel moody and tired, have a hard time getting warm, and experience lowered mental acuity. In addition, soy is high in phytates, an enzyme inhibitor that blocks mineral absorption in the digestive tract. This is why many people experience gas, bloating, cramps, and other digestive upsets after consuming soy. Soy also causes water retention, something I do not want my detoxers to deal with! So, if you're a soy junkie, limit yourself to no more than two servings a week before starting on a cleanse.

REDUCE YOUR SUGAR INTAKE

Sugar is one of the most addictive chemicals on earth. Seriously. I know that you know this! But if you don't, consider a recent study by French scientists that found that in animal trials, rats chose sugar over cocaine every time they were given a choice. Even the rats that were previously addicted to cocaine chose sugar over cocaine! Furthermore, fructose (a form of sugar) fools our brains into thinking we are not full, so we overeat. Because sugar cannot be converted into energy by the mitochondria inside our cells, it is turned into liver fat. It also tampers

MAKE YOUR KITCHEN HEALTH-SUPPORTIVE

One of the easiest ways to create a more health-supportive home is to remove items from your kitchen shelves, fridge, and freezer that don't contribute to your success. The worst of these are packaged foods that contain chemical ingredients of all kinds. Any time you find an item that contains a crazy-sounding, polysyllabic, lab-made chemical, put it in a garbage bag.

Once you've finished, you have a choice regarding that bag of naughty food: You can throw the bag away in a trash can that is not in your home, or give the unopened items to a neighborhood pantry, a homeless shelter, your next-door neighbor, or anyone else who does not live in your space.

If you are feeling energetic, start wiping down your kitchen and tossing out any clutter. A clean, bright, streamlined kitchen is not only a joy to behold, it makes detoxing easier, too.

with blood sugar levels, creating a cycle of cravings—the more sugar you eat, the more you'll crave. The result is insulin resistance (insulin promotes sugar uptake from blood), which leads to chronic metabolic disease, including diabetes and heart disease. Plus, sugar lowers your immune system function and creates puffiness and bloat. You are better off without it, and you must go without it altogether during a cleanse to get the results you want. So, I'm asking you now to start choosing sugar-free snacks and refrain from adding sugar to beverages as you get ready to experience the 7-Day Superfood Cleanse.

CLEAR YOUR KITCHEN

Whenever you do something new or something difficult, you prepare, right? It is the same with doing a cleanse. To set yourself up for success, keep only health-supportive foods in your kitchen. In the days leading up to the 7-Day Superfood Cleanse, refrain from bringing "problem foods" into your kitchen and onto the table—you want to keep your environment as supportive and nurturing as possible.

Now, I'm not saying that you can never have a cookie or an ice cream cone or whatever sweet thing happens to calls out to you; I'm saying that if you really want one of these foods, you'll have to go out (yes, travel!) to get it and then consume whatever it is away from home. Maybe you'll go to the corner store and then sit on a bench and savor that cookie instead of pulling a package out of the cupboard and eating everything in the box. Or maybe you'll go to the local ice cream parlor and get a cone instead of sitting on the sofa at home with a pint of the stuff. You get the idea: You're less likely to abuse food if it requires an effort to get it. Special foods should be special, not everyday staples. This strategy alone will help you enormously on your get-healthy and weight-loss journey.

If you live with others, see if you can get them used to going out for special food treats as well. It will serve everyone's best interests.

TRY A GREEN DRINK!

The best time to try a green drink is now. Right this instant. The second best time is within the next half hour or so. That's why I want you to turn to chapter 4 and take a look at the *Green Drink Blueprints* (pages 54–57). Then I want you to make one for yourself. You can use a blender or a juicer, depending on your preference. Or, if you don't have one of these machines, step out and purchase a bottled green juice—they're easy to find at your local health-food store and most high-quality food stores. Just make sure that your green juice is made without a lot of fruit and contains less than 10 grams of sugar per serving.

For most of us, there's a learning curve when it comes to enjoying green drinks. It takes a bit of experimentation to hit upon just the right combination of ingredients—a blend that contains a taste of something you love and supports your health goals. Luckily, you'll find plenty of superfood ingredients in the *Green Drink Blueprints* to make the process easy and enjoyable. I strongly suggest that you begin to experiment with green drinks such as these before diving into the 7-Day Superfood

Cleanse. I want you to be able to hit the detox ground running, which you will certainly be able to do if you give yourself a bit of time beforehand to literally get a taste of the detox before you begin.

YOUR SOCIAL CALENDAR

Are there good or bad times to detox? I can detox just about any time, even in the middle of a trip to France, during the Christmas holidays, or during periods of major stress. That's because every time I run a group cleanse program, I detox with everyone who participates, so I am used to the process. But that may not be true for you. It's been my experience that most people prefer to detox during a relatively stressless week, when there are no foodie trips or holidays (such as Thanksgiving) or client lunches. If that scenario makes sense to you, take a look at your calendar and choose a week. Then write in big red letters CLEANSE WEEK—KEEP CLEAR! Enjoying a week without heavy work and social commitments will give you the time to reflect, notice what's going on with you, and dive deep into the cleanse.

Having said that, some of you may do better if you detox during a busy work week, where you can pack your food for work, do the cleanse, get your work done, and come home and fall asleep without too much spare time to ruminate. I get that, too. Whichever camp you fall into, please honor it and choose your cleanse week accordingly.

Now that you've begun to prepare your mind, body, and home for the 7-Day Superfood Cleanse, are you ready to get started? In the next chapter, you'll discover how to set up your pantry—which foods to have on hand—and how to use them in the 7-Day Superfood Cleanse. Find out which cleanse plan makes the most sense for your goals (following the Everyday Cleanse Plan for the whole week or substituting days 4 and 6 with the optional, hardcore Quick Cleanse Plan), along with tips on mastering the "cleanse mindset" in order to achieve your goals. Let's go!

HOW IT ALL WORKS

Y OU ARE ALMOST READY TO BEGIN the 7-Day Superfood Cleanse! To make sure you are set up for success in a way that is safe and easy for you—no matter what your goals, needs, and challenges—this chapter gives you everything you need to know in order to dive in deep and have the best possible experience while you are on the 7-Day Superfood Cleanse. Here you'll find out about the two meal plans on which the cleanse is based and which one makes the most sense for you, given your goals. Either way, you'll discover the pivotal role of wise food choices (what you eat), as well as when you eat and how you eat. You'll also learn about lifestyle choices that have nothing at all to do with food but will make the experience of detoxing and staying healthy that much more enjoyable and, ultimately, more successful.

Although it is true that you can do the 7-Day Superfood Cleanse without the information I'm about to share with you, I speak from experience when I say that doing a bit of easy preparation before you start can make your detox so much more effective, easy, and fun. (Incidentally, fun is important—especially when you are making an effort to upgrade your health!) The more you enjoy yourself, the more likely you are to stick to health-supportive behaviors. That's why I put a premium on pleasure throughout the 7-Day Superfood Cleanse.

WISE FOOD CHOICES

Food is the cornerstone of most health-improving programs, and the 7-Day Superfood Cleanse is no exception. What makes it different, however, is the kind of food around which the 7-Day Superfood Cleanse is built. Superfoods, also known as functional foods, medicinal foods, or power foods, are at the core of the cleanse and contain unusually nutrient-dense ingredients that not only help prevent a wide range of health conditions, but can also help restore your health, energy, looks, and mental acuity.

A GOOD, CLEAN SWEAT

During the 7-Day Superfood Cleanse, you'll be stepping up your movement—not to crazy, time-consuming levels, but enough to improve your circulation and do a bit of sweating. Sweating is a good thing: Toxins leave the body in several ways, including perspiration, which is one of the quickest. If your health will allow it, other sweaty activities—from saunas to sex—are encouraged!

Detoxes require that you eat more restrictively than usual. When you remove a large number of ingredients from your diet, however, it's important to take a close look at what you leave in, which is why every meal and snack in the 7-Day Superfood Cleanse is based on a tight roster of nutritionally dense superfoods.

In order to help your body lose bloat, shed weight, and start flushing stored toxins, you must take a break from a host of water-retaining ingredients such as animal products (meat, dairy, eggs), wheat, soy, chemical ingredients, coffee, sugar, and alcohol. Excluding yogurt, cereal, sandwiches, pasta, chicken, beef, fish, and other cleanse no-nos may seem a bit harsh and give you the impression that there will be few foods to enjoy—but the actuality is that there are surprisingly delicious options to be had for every meal of the day, including snacks, on the 7-Day Superfood Cleanse.

Now that you know which unhealthy foods to get rid of while you're preparing to cleanse, it's time to focus on replenishing the shelves in your kitchen, fridge, and freezer with a range of delicious super-food ingredients you'll want to eat and drink while you're actually cleansing.

If you're a takeout lover or a restaurant-goer, or if you travel a lot, you'll still want to take a look at the shopping list—it will be relevant to you, too. And I'm absolutely not going to ask you to cook if you don't want to or don't have the time! I want the 7-Day Superfood Cleanse to be easy and fun for you, so I have not listed every single thing that is good for you. Nor have I listed every single thing that you should avoid. I don't want you to feel overwhelmed by daunting requirements.

THE 7-DAY SUPERFOOD CLEANSE SHOPPING LIST

The items in the list below are things I'd like you to have in your kitchen or that you can easily buy from delis, grocery store salad bars, or restaurants—if you're not a cook or if you travel often. Just be sure that the ingredients are wholesome (see the list of superfoods that starts on page 26). The concentration of phytonutrients, vitamins, minerals, and other goodies, such as fatty acids, amino acids, healthy fats, and fiber, in these foods will help support your health and keep you energized and focused while you clear your head and shed pounds.

Having said that: Flexibility is important! Take a look at the shopping list, then stock up on the things that you'd like to have at home, or pull out the restaurant menus you use frequently to order food (or look them up online). Study them a bit and see which items will do a good job of supporting your cleanse. Or do a mental walk-through of your favorite deli, takeout joint, or salad bar. The idea is to get acquainted now with your options. Feel free to take a look at the Resources section (page 171) to help you find healthy superfood options if you live in an area where they are difficult to find locally.

Then there are plenty of optional foods you can add in. You'll find a list on page 28, but remember, these are truly optional, so don't feel like you need to run out and get them all. You probably have a number of these in your kitchen right now! These everyday favorites make eating more fun, so if you're up for adventure, now's a great time to try a few that are new to you.

NOTE: If you do not like an item on the shopping list, do not buy it. If you are allergic to something I have listed, do not buy it. If you have a health condition that is aggravated by something on the list, do not buy it.

- MIXED SALAD GREENS, ARUGULA, OR OTHER DARK SALAD GREENS: 1–2 pounds
- SPINACH for use in green drinks (which encompass both green smoothies and green juices; pages 54–57 for recipes): 1–2 pounds
- ROMAINE for use in green drinks: 1 pound
- FRESH HERBS, such as parsley, cilantro, dill, and so on for use in green drinks (fresh herbs are rich in chlorophyll, phytonutrients, vitamin K, protein, and are tremendously detoxifying): 1 or 2 bunches
- KALE, COLLARDS, CHARD, OR OTHER GREEN LEAFY VEGETABLES for use in green drinks: 1–2 pounds
- CUCUMBERS: 7 or 8
- COCONUT WATER for green drinks: 1 or 2 boxes or bottles
- LEMONS OR LIMES: 10 or more large
- APPLE CIDER VINEGAR, preferably a health food store variety that contains the "mother," a webby-looking clot (sorry—I know how gross that sounds) floating around near the bottom of the bottle: 1 bottle
- YOUR FAVORITE RAW SNACKING VEGGIES, such as avocado, cucumber, bell peppers, broccoli, carrots, tomatoes, jicama, snow/snap peas, or any others that you like
- HUMMUS, SALSA, AND/OR VEGAN BEAN DIP: 1 or more containers
- VEGAN VEGGIE SOUPS (companies such as Pacific and Imagine have good options); look for varieties free from dairy, soy, and gluten that are made with tomato, pumpkin, winter squash, sweet potato, red pepper, and broccoli (or other cruciferous veggies) because these superfood ingredients are dense in nutrients: several boxed (aseptic boxes)
- CANNED OR DRIED LEGUMES, such as black beans, red kidney beans, cannellini beans, pinto beans, black-eyed

peas, mung beans, lentils, split peas, and other legumes (all of which are nourishing superfoods!) if you like to cook: 5–7 cans (or 2–2.5 pounds dried) of your favorite

- NUTS AND/OR SEEDS, such as walnuts, pistachios, Brazil nuts, cashews, almonds, pumpkin seeds (look for the green, hull-less pepitas), and sunflower seeds (peanuts often contain a microscopic mold, which is why I don't call for them or peanut products on the detox; if you're a peanut lover, use this week as an opportunity to explore other fabulous nuts and seeds): 1 or 2 pounds of your favorite
- ALMOND, CASHEW, HAZELNUT, OR SUNFLOWER SEED BUTTER: 1 or more jars
- QUINOA (if you don't cook, try frozen premade quinoa or grain mixes available in the freezer section—just run hot water on them and you have a meal): 1 or 2 pounds
- BROWN RICE, MILLET, OR AMARANTH (if you don't cook, try frozen premade rice or grain mixes available in the freezer section— just run hot water on them and you have a meal): 1 pound
- BLACK TEA (such as English breakfast or Earl Grey) and HERBAL TEA (try one of the detox teas out there; most herbal tea companies—from Yogi to Celestial Seasonings brands—make a detox or "cleansing" tea): 1 or more boxes of your favorite
- COLD-PRESSED EXTRA VIRGIN OLIVE OIL AND/OR COCONUT OIL: 8-ounce or larger bottle
- CHIA SEED (WHOLE) (I love those from Health Warrior, but you can also try Navitas Naturals, AZ Chia, or whatever brand is available at your local health food store): 1 pound
- SUPERFOOD VEGGIES, such as avocado, beets, bell peppers (any color), cabbage, chard, collards, kale, spinach,

sweet potato, tomatoes, winter squash, and so on: as many of your favorites as you think you'll eat

- YOUR FAVORITE EVERYDAY VEGGIES that aren't necessarily superfoods but are important for your health nonetheless, such as asparagus, artichokes, celery, celeriac, jicama, radishes, and so on: as many as you think you'll eat

OPTIONAL FOODS

These foods are optional, so don't feel that you need to run out and get all of them, but they will make eating more fun:

- Any of the optional extras found in the *Green Drink Blueprints* (pages 54–57)
- Any of the ingredients called for in the *Winter Pink Drink* (pages 59–60), or *Summer Watermelon Detox Smoothie* (page 61)
- Any of the ingredients called for in any of the recipes in chapters 4–10
- 1 head of garlic, onion, and/or bunch of scallions
- 1 large knob of ginger
- SPICES AND FLAVORINGS, including curry, hot sauce, fish sauce, jerk paste, organic soy sauce, and so on (spices and hot sauces are considered superfoods because they strengthen the immune system, allowing it to help rid the body of toxins; choose whatever spices you like, knowing that you are helping your body cleanse itself naturally)
- SELTZER WATER to make fun beverages
- VINEGARS AND/OR NUT OILS (almond, hazelnut, pumpkin seed, pistachio, walnut), for drizzling over salads
- PREMADE NATURAL SALAD DRESSINGS (no Wishbone!) for drizzling over salads
- PRETTY FLOWERS for your dining table, kitchen counter, or desk, as a reminder of how special you are

GETTING INTO THE CLEANSE MINDSET

As you move through the 7-Day Superfood Cleanse, I want you to think: Ease. Grace. Flow. Find a way to fit the detox into your current life instead of twisting your schedule and yourself into a pretzel in order to "do this detox thing." I assure you, a detox can happen successfully in even the busiest of lives. You'll see! The following tips may help you get through the week.

- Read this book all the way through before you begin the 7-Day Superfood Cleanse.
- Check your work and social calendar and choose a week that will work best for you. If you are someone who eats out of boredom, don't choose a slow week to do the cleanse—you'll be tempted to give in to unhealthy eating anytime things get tedious. If you are a stress eater, go for a calm, low-pressure week, so you won't be tempted to raid the office vending machine for something sweet to calm your nerves.
- If you can, steer clear of holidays, big events, and travel while you're doing a cleanse. A cleanse takes you out of your routine, and trying to do a cleanse at those times can mean frustration and guilt—neither of which is going to help you lose weight or get healthy!
- Study the shopping list that starts on page 26 and see what you'll need to stock your kitchen.
- Clear your kitchen of foods that won't help you succeed with the cleanse.
- Peruse both meal plans for the 7-Day Superfood Cleanse before detoxing, and look at the recipes in chapters 4–10 to identify anything that you'd like to try.
- Decide if you want to tell your friends and other loved ones that you are detoxing. Most of us have friends or family who are terrific cheerleaders, but you may also have loved ones who try to sabotage your efforts anytime you try to improve your health (or any other part of your life, for that matter). So I will give you the same advice I give my clients. It's the only time I ever refer to

a religious text, and the quote comes from Matthew 7:6 in the King James Bible: "Give not that which is holy unto the dogs, neither cast ye your pearls before swine, lest they trample them under their feet, and turn again and rend you." In other words, be wise about the people you choose to tell about your latest plan for self-improvement!

- Buy some great books and self-care products and stock up on uplifting movies. During a cleanse you are giving your body and your health a fresh start—the perfect time to enjoy positive, empowering movies and books.
- When you become overwhelmed, address the issue immediately. If this is the case, I advise you to do one thing: Breathe. Just breathe. Anytime you change a habit it's natural to feel over-whelmed. But the 7-Day Superfood Cleanse is also super easy.

THE SLEEP-DETOX EQUATION

During the 7-Day Superfood Cleanse I encourage you to get as much sleep as you can—at least 8 hours if possible—but if you can get more (or fit in a daily nap of any length), please do. When you sleep, your body repairs muscle tissue, regenerates new cells, consolidates daytime memories, flushes toxins into the urinary tract and large intestines for excretion, and releases hormones that regulate growth and appetite. The more sleep you get, the more opportunity you give your body to do these things—and the less chance you'll have to engage in health-harmful activities such as late-night eating and drinking. In addition, a fatigued body is more likely to crave sugar and other carbohydrates and caffeine, making it a struggle to stick to a cleanse (or any other healthy eating) program. So, throughout the 7-Day Superfood Cleanse, I'll remind you to get plenty of rest! Please give yourself this gift. Your reinvigorated, slimmer body will thank you, too.

Just do the best you can. During the week you're on the cleanse, you may make a non-detoxing food choice once in a while. So be it. "Once in a while" is better than constantly making non-detoxing food choices.

THE 7-DAY SUPERFOOD CLEANSE MEAL PLANS

The 7-Day Superfood Cleanse is based on two meal plans, both of which include nutrient-dense superfoods to ensure that your body is deeply nourished even though you may be eating less food than you would in an ordinary week.

1. THE EVERYDAY CLEANSE PLAN is the engine of the 7-Day Superfood Cleanse. This mixed whole food and liquid meal plan gives you the most choices for every meal and snack of the day, every day of the week. It is designed to help your body shed toxins and trapped water weight, jump-start weight loss, and leave you feeling light, energetic, focused, and free of unhealthy-food cravings.

2. THE QUICK CLEANSE PLAN is strictly optional—use it only on days 4 and 6 if you want to kick things up a notch. This meal plan consists mainly of liquids and is designed to give your digestive system the break it needs to release deeply held toxins and flush out large amounts of water weight thoroughly and quickly. The Quick Cleanse Plan should be followed for no more than one day at a time and should be used *only* on days 4 and 6 of the 7-Day Superfood Cleanse.

Are you ready? Here's all I ask: Do your best. Your best will improve each day and your body will thank you for sticking with it.

NOTE: If you are on a special diet, please make sure that your food selections from the Everyday Cleanse Plan and/or the Quick Cleanse Plan agree with it. Be sure to discuss the meal plan you intend to use on the 7-Day Superfood Cleanse with your health care provider before you begin. I want you to feel great this week!

THE EVERYDAY CLEANSE PLAN
FOR DAYS 1–7

UPON WAKING / BEFORE BREAKFAST

Start each day with a glass of room-temperature water. Increasing your fresh water intake may seem counterintuitive, but it actually encourages your body to let go of stored water weight. Adding a splash of lemon juice or vinegar helps fight physical and mental fatigue, encourages your body to become alkalized (so it can flush toxins), and helps squelch the carbohydrate cravings that can make detoxes difficult for so many people. Herbal tea, another cleanse food, is used during the week for many of the same reasons.

THROUGHOUT THE DAY

Sip water throughout the day. Feel free to add lemon or lime juice, apple cider vinegar, or cucumber slices. Keep water with you at all times to make it easy to stay hydrated.

BREAKFAST

Both *Green Drink* recipes (the blender version and the juicer version) in chapter 5, "Breakfast" (page 69), are appropriate for the Everyday Cleanse Plan and the Quick Cleanse plan.

Breakfast consists of:

- A glass of water (maybe with a splash of lemon juice or apple cider vinegar)
- A low-sugar, superfood-filled green drink, rich in phytonutrients. The cornerstone of the 7-Day Superfood Cleanse, this green drink ensures that you start your day with all the nutrients you'll need to feel energetic and focused, while supporting detoxification, strengthening your immune system, and alkalizing your system so that you won't experience carbohydrate cravings. You'll find easy-to-follow blueprints for making and customizing green drinks on pages 54–57, but store-bought, premade, or fresh-pressed green drinks work just as well.

CHEW, CHEW, CHEW!

Would you believe that the average American chews his or her food just eight times? If you don't believe me, just watch someone eat, or eat in front of a mirror and watch yourself. Underchewing wreaks havoc on your body's digestive and detoxification abilities.

Underchewing matters because digestion begins not in the stomach but in the mouth, with chewing. Chewing leads to smooth digestion and greater assimilation of nutrients by initiating the release of digestive enzymes that break down food.

Chewing helps make oils, proteins, vitamins, minerals, and other nutrients available for maximum absorption. Mixing food with saliva until the food liquefies helps release its full nutritional value, and because digestion becomes so efficient when you chew your food thoroughly, your body will begin to feel wonderfully light. Chewing your food thoroughly is an easy way to help your body fully digest and assimilate the nutrients it needs to help flush out toxins.

Starting with the next snack or meal, chew each mouthful of food at least thirty times. You will feel ridiculous doing this. But try it anyway. Get in the habit of putting down your utensils between bites and focus on chewing, chewing, chewing.

- OPTIONAL: If you'd like a more protein-rich drink, add 1 or 2 tablespoons of nut butter, up to ¼ cup of nuts or seeds, or a scoop of non-soy plant protein powder to your green drink. (For more information about this, see chapter 5. Or simply enjoy munching on a handful of nuts or seeds with your green drink.
- ADDITIONAL OPTION: 1 cup of black or green tea or herbal tea, unsweetened. If you'd like to add a splash of coconut milk, go ahead.

• IF YOU ARE ABSOLUTELY STARVING, feel free to enjoy a cup of last night's dinner leftovers (see chapter 8 for all dinner recipes), such as *Simple Tomato Soup* (page 121) or *Nutty Kale Salad* (page 126), or a cup of any of the lunch recipes in chapter 6 with your green drink. Try *Grain or Bean Salad Blueprint* (page 80) or *Mexicali Quinoa Pilaf* (page 84). Be creative!

EXFOLIATE, STIMULATE, EXFOLIATE

To set up your body for accelerated detoxing, try this deceptively easy, non-food-related trick to help your body shed toxins and stored fat quickly and easily. It's called skin brushing. Use it every day while you're detoxing for the best results. Here's how:

- Use a hot towel, a dry (or wet or soapy) body brush, a commercial body scrub, a loofah, or a rough washcloth to vigorously brush your skin.
- Start at your feet and brush upward, toward the heart. Then tackle your arms, starting with your fingers and working your way up. You can do your chest and neck last. Brushing your face is optional.

Brushing your skin helps improve blood circulation throughout the body and stimulates your lymphatic system, which also helps remove toxins from the body. Brushing your skin also gets rid of dead skin cells—which contain toxins, especially if you've been on a detox program, and keeps those toxins from being reabsorbed into the body. Removing dead skin cells gives the body a clear, unencumbered path for the removal of the next wave of toxins your body wants to eliminate through the skin.

How often should you brush your skin? Daily, if you can—or at least when you remember. Whatever you do, your body will appreciate it!

All recipes in chapter 7, "Snacks" (page 98), are appropriate for the Everyday Cleanse Plan. Snacks ensure that you'll never go hungry. Happily, there are lots of options to enjoy mid-morning and in the mid-afternoon—or whenever your energy and resolve start to lag.

NOTE: Options for midmorning and midafternoon snacks are the same; they can be savory, sweet, hot, cold, crunchy, or smooth, depending on your taste. And, depending on the meal plan you've chosen for the 7-Day Superfood Cleanse, your midmorning or midafternoon snack can be solid or liquid.

- Good snack options, which you'll find in chapter 7, include: *Raw Zucchini Hummus* (page 110), *White Bean Dip* (page 112), *Avocado-Coconut Dip* (page 113), *Easy Pumpkin Protein Dip* (page 113), and *Garlicky Kale and Spinach Dip* (page 114)
- *Baked Kale Chips* (page 107), *Coconut Chips* (page 105), and *Salt and Vinegar Kale Chips* (page 108) provide crave-worthy crunch to go along with hearty and sustaining dips (such as those mentioned above and in chapter 7)—or you can use store-bought kale chips that do not contain soy, dairy, or wheat. Coconut chips are also available in some stores. Be sure to buy a brand that does not contain any added chemical ingredients.
- To further satisfy your cravings for crunch, you can also opt for a handful of *Roasted Coconut Chickpeas* (page 106) or nuts (about ¼ cup—but don't stress if you eat more; you'll still be detoxing).
- If you're unable to make your own dip, try store-bought hummus, bean dip, or guacamole. Just be sure they are made without dairy.
- 2 tablespoons of nut butter—such as almond or cashew—also makes a fine dip for veggies.
- Have a cup of soup. Use any recipe for soup in chapter 8, or use a premade dairy-free, wheat-free, pureed vegetable soup.
- *Chia Fresca* (page 100) or *Chia Pudding* (page 101), also in chapter 7, is soothing and filling as a mid-morning or mid-afternoon snack.
- If you have chosen the Quick Cleanse Plan for days 4 and 6 of the

7-Day Superfood Cleanse and want a liquid-only snack, you'll enjoy any of these refreshing drinks: *Summer Watermelon Detox Smoothie* (page 61), *Winter Pink Drink* (pages 59–60), *Carrot Lassi* (page 62), *Citrus Zinger* (page 62), *Coconut Cooler* (page 63), *Key Lime–Coconut Frappé* (page 64), *Lemon Water* (page 63), or *Lemon Ginger Detox Drink* (page 64).

- Enjoy one or two cups of any of the detox teas in chapter 4 (page 65), and severala cups of herbal tea, your choice, brewed with a store-bought herbal tea bag, or a cup of *Classic Lemon-Ginger Tea* (page 66) is another good option.

LUNCH

Lunch is the day's largest meal. Eating the bulk of your calories midday allows your body to utilize them fully, so you don't store calories (which leads to weight gain). You'll find a range of sit-down and brownbag lunch recipes, plus takeout suggestions in chapter 6 (page 76).

- All recipes in chapter 6, "Lunch," are appropriate for the Everyday Cleanse Plan.
- Any of the recipes in the Complete Meal Options section of chapter 6 (page 77) make perfect one-dish lunches. These include the: *Grain or Bean Salad Blueprint* (page 80—a great way to create your own protein-rich detox dish!), *Quinoa Superfood Salad* (page 81), *Black-Eyed Pea Salad* (page 83), *Gingered Millet with Japanese Veggies* (page 82), *Black Rice Salad* (page 85), and *Mexicali Quinoa Pilaf* (page 84).
- If you're traveling or don't have the time to make your own grain-veggie-legume dish from scratch, you can pick one up from a salad bar, health food store, or restaurant.
- Have any of the recipes in the Grains section (page 86) served with one or two of the recipes in the Veggie section (page 91).
- Grain dishes include: *Millet with Roasted Sunflower Seeds* (page 87), *Brown Rice Medley* (page 86), *Coconut Quinoa* (page 90), and *Coconut Brown Rice* (page 89).
- Veggie recipes include: *Side Salad Blueprint* (page 92), *Braised*

ABOUT EVENING COCKTAILS
AND OTHER ALCOHOLIC BEVERAGES

Alcohol (enjoyed in moderation, of course!) is an important part of many of our lives. Mine, too. But for the next 7 days, do your absolute best to avoid alcohol. The liver and the rest of the body work hard to metabolize and shunt alcohol out of your system, so it doesn't make sense to add toxins, such as alcohol, to our bodies during a detox. So for now, go dry. Break out the other bubbly (seltzer), put it in a sexy glass, dress it up with lemon or lime, and make a toast to your health. Skoal!

Coconut Spinach and Chickpeas with Lemon (page 93), *Roasted Veggies in Coconut Oil* (page 94), *Classic Greens* (page 95), *Indian Greens* (page 96), and *Sautéed Broccoli Rabe* (page 97). Or, if it's more convenient, you can grab a takeout vegan veggie curry, a bowl of vegetarian chili, or a stir-fry served over millet. And of course you can order something similar from a restaurant if you're on the road or don't have time to make one of these dishes from scratch.

• Enjoy a cup of herbal tea, your choice, brewed with a store-bought herbal tea bag, or a cup of *Classic Lemon-Ginger Tea* (page 66).

DINNER

Dinner, during a detox, is a light affair that's easy to digest and ensures that your body can do the deep work of cleansing while you sleep. Typically, it consists of a soup and/or salad. To make sure that you are thoroughly satisfied with this light meal, I've developed recipes that are nutrient-dense, filling, and flavorful. In chapter 8, you'll also find good suggestions for takeout and restaurant dinners that work well for light dinners.

• All recipes in chapter 8, "Dinner" (page 115), are appropriate for the Everyday Cleanse Plan.

- While following the Everyday Cleanse Plan, you can enjoy either soup or salad each evening, or have both! It's your choice.
- Soup recipes in chapter 8 include: *Dinner Soup Blueprint* (page 117), which allows you to have fun creating your own detox-supportive soups, such as *Spicy Pumpkin Coconut Bisque* (page 118), *Superfood Beet Soup* (page 119), *Carrot Soup* (page 120), and *Simple Tomato Soup* (page 121). You also have the option to go with a premade vegan soup, whether you buy it fresh from the store, enjoy it in a restaurant, or have it delivered to your home.
- Salad recipes in chapter 8 include: *Dinner Salad Blueprint* (page 123), which allows you to create a fabulous detox-friendly salad using your choice of ingredients, such as *Chopped Avocado Coconut Salad* (my favorite; page 124), *Celeriac and Beet Salad* (page 125), *Nutty Kale Salad* (page 126), and a host of tasty homemade cleanse-worthy salad dressings. Of course you can pick up a premade salad or order one at a restaurant, if you're on the road or don't have the time to make one.
- Enjoy a cup of herbal tea, your choice, brewed with a store-bought herbal tea bag, or a cup of *Classic Lemon-Ginger Tea* (page 66).

IS IT OKAY TO SNACK BEFORE GOING TO BED?

For many people, the time after dinner and before bedtime is notorious for snacking. Unfortunately, you can't snack after dinner and fully detoxify, nor can you lose weight quickly if you're eating before bedtime. If you really feel like you need a little something before you hit the sack, try one of these:
- One or more cups of unsweetened herbal tea
- One cup of warm vegetable broth
- Seltzer or mineral water with a slice of lemon, lime, or cucumber
- Regular tap or bottled water with a slice of lemon, lime, or cucumber

THE QUICK CLEANSE PLAN:
AN OPTIONAL, HARDCORE PLAN
FOR DAYS 4 AND 6

While everyone will enjoy the meals in the Everyday Cleanse Plan, some of you may choose to dive into an accelerated cleanse to achieve your goals. Liquid-heavy and designed to be followed for no more than one day at a time (for a total of two non-consecutive days—that is, days 4 and 6 of the Everyday Cleanse Plan), this hardcore plan will increase weight and water loss while flushing toxins from your digestive system even more quickly than the Everyday Cleanse Plan.

Although it is more restrictive, the Quick Cleanse Plan allows you to consume food at regular intervals during the day, but it does require that you decrease your intake of excess protein and drink more liquid-based foods in order to give your digestion a bit of a rest so that your body can spend more energy on detoxing. The plan is still easy to follow, however, even if you have a busy week or are traveling. Simply follow the Everyday Cleanse Plan, except on days 4 and 6, when you will use *only* the recipes below.

BEFORE BREAKFAST/UPON WAKING

- Drink a large glass of lukewarm water (not cold!) with a squirt (about 1 teaspoon) of lemon or lime juice or a splash of apple cider vinegar.

THROUGHOUT THE DAY

- Sip water throughout the day. Feel free to add lemon or lime juice, apple cider vinegar, or cucumber slices. Keep water with you at all times to make it easy to stay hydrated.

BREAKFAST

- Drink one glass of room temperature water with a splash of lemon or lime juice or apple cider vinegar.
- Enjoy one *Green Drink* (pages 54–57). Per the optional add-in directions, add some protein to the drink, such as a handful of nuts,

1 or 2 tablespoons of nut butter, or a scoop of protein powder.

- OPTIONAL ADDITION: 1 cup of black or green or herbal tea, unsweetened. If you'd like to add a splash of coconut milk, go ahead.

OPTIONAL MID-MORNING SNACKS

Choose as many of these as you like for a mid-morning snack—or any time you need to re-energize and keep focused:

- One cup of herbal tea, your choice, or a cup of *Classic Lemon-Ginger Tea* (page 66)
- *Chia Fresca* (page 100) or *Chia Pudding* (page 101)
- Any of these refreshing drinks: *Summer Watermelon Detox Smoothie* (page 61), *Winter Pink Drink* (pages 59–60), *Carrot Lassi* (page 62), *Citrus Zinger* (page 62), *Coconut Cooler* (page 63), *Key Lime–Coconut Frappé* (page 64), *Lemon Water* (page 63), *Lemon Ginger Detox Drink* (page 64), or any of the herbal or detox teas in chapter 4 (page 65), or a cup of herbal tea brewed with a store-bought herbal tea bag.

LUNCH

You'll discover, happily, when you're on the Quick Cleanse Plan that lunch on days 4 and 6 has a bit more substance than a green drink, smoothie, or soup. A sturdy midday meal will give your body the calories it needs to stay healthy, while giving you the energy you need to get through the afternoon and stay focused.

- Any of the Complete Meal Option recipes in chapter 6 make excellent one-dish lunches. These include the *Grain or Bean Salad Blueprint* (page 80—a great way to create your own protein-rich detox dish!), *Quinoa Superfood Salad* (page 81), *Black-Eyed Pea Salad* (page 83), *Gingered Millet with Japanese Veggies* (page 82), *Black Rice Salad* (page 85), and *Mexicali Quinoa Pilaf* (page 84). If you're traveling or don't have the time to make your own grain-veggie-legume dish from scratch, you can pick one up from a salad bar, health food store, or restaurant.
- Any of the dishes in the Grains section served with one or two

of the recipes in the Veggie section. Grain dishes include *Millet with Roasted Sunflower Seeds* (page 87), *Brown Rice Medley* (page 86), *Coconut Quinoa* (page 90), and *Coconut Brown Rice* (page 89). Veggie recipes include *Side Salad Blueprint* (page 92), *Braised Coconut Spinach and Chickpeas with Lemon* (page 93), *Roasted Veggies in Coconut Oil* (page 94), *Classic Greens* (page 95), *Indian Greens* (page 96), and *Sautéed Broccoli Rabe* (page 97). Or, if it's more convenient, you can grab a takeout vegan veggie curry, a bowl of vegetarian chili, or a stir-fry served over millet. And of course you can order something similar from a restaurant if you're on the road or don't have time to make one of these dishes from scratch.

- Have a *Summer Watermelon Detox Smoothie* (page 61), *Winter Pink Drink* (pages 59–60), *Carrot Lassi* (page 62), *Citrus Zinger* (page 62), *Coconut Cooler* (page 63), *Key Lime–Coconut Frappé* (page 64), *Lemon Water* (page 63), or *Lemon Ginger Detox Drink* (page 64).
- Enjoy a cup of herbal tea of your choice, brewed with a store-bought herbal tea bag, or a cup of *Classic Lemon-Ginger Tea* (page 66).

OPTIONAL MID-AFTERNOON SNACKS

Choose as many of these as you like for a mid-afternoon snack—or any time you need to re-energize and keep focused.
- Seltzer with lemon or lime juice
- *Chia Fresca* (page 100) or *Chia Pudding* (page 101)
- *Summer Watermelon Detox Smoothie* (page 61), *Winter Pink Drink* (pages 59–60), *Carrot Lassi* (page 62), *Citrus Zinger* (page 62), *Coconut Cooler* (page 63), *Key Lime–Coconut Frappé* (page 64), *Lemon Water* (page 63), or *Lemon Ginger Detox Drink* (page 64).
- One or two cups of any of the detox teas in chapter 4 (page 65) or a cup of herbal tea brewed with a store-bought herbal tea bag.

DINNER

Feel free to enjoy either a drink or soup, or have one of each if you're really hungry.
- *Green Drink* (pages 54–57), *Summer Watermelon Detox Smoothie* (page 61), or *Winter Pink Drink* made without protein (pages 59–60), are good choices. Other recipes for green drinks, smoothies, teas, and additional beverages, all of which may be enjoyed for dinner if you are following the Quick Cleanse Plan, may be found in chapter 4 (page 39).
- Vegan soup recipes in chapter 8 include *Dinner Soup Blueprint* (page 117), which gives you a base for creating your own detox-supportive soups, such as *Spicy Pumpkin Coconut Bisque* (page 118), *Superfood Beet Soup* (page 119), *Carrot Soup* (page 120), and

Simple Tomato Soup (page 121). You also have the option to have a premade vegan soup, whether you buy it fresh from the store, enjoy it in a restaurant, or have it delivered to your home.

OPTIONAL POST-DINNER SNACKS

Help yourself to as much as you like of these two postprandial snacks:
- Herbal tea of your choice, or a cup of *Classic Lemon-Ginger Tea* (page 66).
- Glass of seltzer or water

WHAT HAPPENS NEXT

In chapter 4 (page 45) you'll discover the health and slimming benefits of green drinks—which include smoothies and juices—used in the Everyday Cleanse Plan as well as the Quick Cleanse Plan, so please make sure to get to know them! You'll find plenty of ways to personalize green drinks, depending on your health, personal preferences, and what you have on hand in the kitchen. I'll even give you some store-bought options if you can't make your own green drinks, along with recipes for several other delicious, cleanse-friendly superfood drinks that you can use no matter which meal plan you happen to be following.

THE DETOX BREATH

Of course, you already know how to breathe, but do you know how to take a "detox breath" and why mastering this method of deep breathing can make you feel healthier and more energized? Read on!

When your body is freshly oxygenated, wounds heal faster, your metabolism runs more efficiently, and you feel energized, calm, focused, mentally sharp, intuitive, creative, and productive. If you're looking for an easy way to nab that feeling, you're in luck.

Just take a breath—but not just any old kind of breath: Take a full-bodied, deep-belly breath—so deep that your abdomen expands and the lowest lobes of your lungs are inflated with oxygen.

At first, this may feel strange. That's because most folks go through their days breathing shallowly, at the very upper portion of their lungs. You'll feel a lot healthier and focused if you send oxygen to the nethermost regions of your lungs. Here's how:

- Sit or stand up straight with your chin up. Open up your rib cage by comfortably positioning your shoulders back.
- At first it can help to have a prompt that shows you how deeply you are breathing. Rest one palm gently on your belly, then slowly and smoothly inhale deeply through your nose. Keep inhaling! You want to see your belly push your hand outward.
- Now hold your breath. Hold it. Hold it. Hold it! When you're ready, slowly exhale through your mouth. Inhale through your nose, exhale through your mouth.
- Repeat five times.

Do you feel the energy-rich oxygen flowing through you? Breathe like this regularly and after a week you'll even notice a fresh glow to your skin!

4

GREEN DRINKS, SMOOTHIES, AND OTHER DETOX DRINKS

D RINKS ARE AN IMPORTANT PART of a detox.

When people talk about detoxes or cleanses, the ever-popular liquid fast often springs to mind. This old-fashioned regimen involves drinking—just drinking—your calories for a specific amount of time. More severe liquid fasts are limited to just water with lemon and maybe a bit of cayenne and honey. Weight loss is at the heart of these often-dangerous liquid fasts, although many people undertake them for spiritual reasons or under supervision of their healthcare provider to help heal a specific health condition.

Before continuing, it's important to reiterate: The 7-Day Superfood Cleanse is not a liquid fast. It does, however, include a lot of drinks simply because they are a great way to give the digestive system (specifically the large intestine) a rest, so that your body's energy can be used for detoxing. Drinks fill you up so you don't feel like snacking, and they deliver a large volume of nutrients to your body almost instantly. I am nothing if not realistic: Are you really going to eat a pound of

A GREEN DRINK CAVEAT

If you have a health condition and are on a special diet, please use veggies that are "safe" for you. For instance, if you can't eat kale, then please do not use it in your green drink! Chop up some green beans or snow peas instead—if they agree with you. If romaine gives you cramps, then use something else. If cucumber makes you burp, then leave it out. The bottom line: Don't be slavish about following any blueprint for a green drink if the ingredients are not safe for you.

GREEN DRINKS AND KIDNEY STONES

Kidney stones are hard deposits composed of minerals and salts that form inside the kidneys. The smaller ones are passed—painfully!—during urination. If you have a history of kidney stones, your healthcare provider may suggest that you lower your intake of oxalate-containing foods. Oxalates are naturally occurring substances found in many foods, and they can cause kidney stones in people who are prone to them. If you are one of these individuals, you don't have to give up green drinks. You simply need to stick to low-oxalate ingredients and avoid high-oxalate foods. Fortunately, this is easy to do.

According to the Glickman Urological and Kidney Institute at the Cleveland Clinic, many foods contain some amount of oxalates, yet only nine foods are known to increase kidney stone formation: beets (including the leaves) and beet relatives, such as chard; spinach; rhubarb; strawberries; nuts; chocolate; tea; wheat bran; and some beans. That leaves you with plenty of other ingredients to use when making your green drinks!

---

raw broccoli, a few sprigs of parsley, a lemon, and two celery stalks for breakfast? I doubt it. However, you can easily take in all of these super beneficial ingredients in a single drink!

In this chapter, I give you some of my favorite recipes for a variety of beverages. These are the cleansing, detoxing drinks I recommend again and again in this book as well as to clients in my private practice. The first recipes you'll find here are the *Green Drink Blueprints*, customizable "recipes" that show you how to make your own green drink using healthy ingredients that you like. The flexibility of the 7-Day Superfood Cleanse ensures that you will be able to customize, enjoy, and benefit from the detoxing power of green drinks, regardless of your personal tastes or health challenges.

In addition to the *Green Drink Blueprints*, which are indeed the cornerstone of the 7-Day Superfood Cleanse, you'll find plenty of other recipes for optional snack-time drinks, such as the *Winter Pink Drink* (pages 59–60), *Summer Watermelon Detox Smoothie* (page 61), and *Carrot Lassi* (page 62). You'll also discover the benefits of herbal teas—the detox variety and "regular" non-detox herbal teas—and how easy (and economical) it is to make herbal tea recipes whenever you want them. Herbal tea is always on the menu during the 7-Day Superfood Cleanse: Enjoy it with breakfast, as a snack, or as a delicious way to quell nighttime eating. The herbs and spices in these teas are rich in anti-inflammatory compounds, as well as phytochemicals that encourage the body to release trapped toxins. And detox formulas have the added benefit of containing one or more ingredients that encourage the body to quickly flush trapped fluids and banish bloat.

Go ahead and drink up!

THE GREEN DRINK, CORNERSTONE OF THE CLEANSE

The green drink is a non-negotiable component of the 7-Day Superfood Cleanse. If you've read chapter 3, which explains how to use the two detox meal plans in the 7-Day Superfood Cleanse, you will have noted that having a green drink is required every single morning. Of course, you can have more than one (or an additional green drink in the afternoon or evening), if you like. The green drink is filled with superfood ingredients to help nourish you, repair your looks, recharge your energy, jump-start weight loss, and flush trapped water weight and toxins from your system. The beauty of the green drink is that it can easily be made in a blender or juicer (whichever is most convenient). You can also buy green drinks from a juice bar or health food shop, or as fresh-pressed, bottled juice.

WHY ARE GREEN DRINKS SO IMPORTANT?

Green drinks are an essential component of the 7-Day Superfood Cleanse because they alkalize the body and squash cravings for carbohydrates. Why is being alkaline such a big deal? It's the most efficient, healthiest place for you to be, where all of your bodily functions—including metabolism—are running at their best.

Do you remember high school chemistry, when you learned about acidic and alkaline pH balances? If you slept through that lesson, here's a refresher: pH stands for potential hydrogen. The body uses hydrogen to help keep its cells hydrated, eliminate toxins and waste, transport nutrients to cells throughout the body, lubricate joints, and help the immune system fight off microbes. Hydrogen also helps the body create energy and protects it from free radical damage, which causes premature aging.

The pH scale is how we measure the concentration of hydrogen ions within an object, including your body. The pH scale ranges from 1 to 14, with 7 considered neutral. A pH less than 7 is said to be acidic. A pH greater than 7 is alkaline. The human body's ideal pH is slightly alkaline—7.30–7.45. This is the sweet spot, the environment where the body's metabolic, enzymatic, immunologic, and repair mechanisms function most efficiently, cravings are low, energy is high, sleep is good, mental acuity is strong, and so on. If the body veers into territory that's too acidic (anything below pH 7), it tries to create a protective buffer to neutralize the acids. It creates this by stealing alkaline minerals (such as potassium, sodium, magnesium, and calcium) from your vital organs, teeth, and bones. The results of being acidic can be fatigue, high blood pressure, kidney stones, poor immune system function, premature aging, osteoporosis, joint pain, muscle aches, mood swings, lack of focus, slow digestion and elimination, bloating, skin conditions, yeast infections, fungal infections, obesity, slow metabolism, and inability to lose weight.

If you're interested, you can test your pH levels regularly. Simply purchase some strips of litmus paper from your local pharmacy and dip one of the strips into your saliva or urine each morning.

So, have your eyes glazed over yet? This may be the easiest way to wrap your head around the alkaline issue: Have an alkalizing green drink every morning! My clients love the way these nutrient-packed elixirs make them feel (and look)—and, hopefully, so will you!

MAKING GREEN DRINKS WORK FOR YOU

Before we dive into the blueprints (yes, they're really more like blueprints than hard-and-fast recipes), there are a few things you should know about it. For one thing, there isn't a whole lot of fruit going on. I mention this for those of you who are currently making green drinks and smoothies with a banana, mango, blueberries, and so on. I love fruit as much as the next person, but to detox quickly and thoroughly, it's best to leave out fruit—and the fruit sugar that comes with it. Having said that, taste is important: I really do want your green drink to be palatable, otherwise you may not drink it. But, since we're moving fast (this is a 7-day cleanse, after all), I also want your green drinks to do what they are supposed to do for you during the detox. Try some of these tips to make your drinks more appetizing:

- Use coconut water. Coconut water contains electrolytes and minerals, making it a replacement for any needed moisture as your body flushes out trapped, bloat-causing fluid during the cleanse. Once you're off the cleanse, I hope you keep up your morning green drinks! If, after your cleanse, you just can't stomach a green drink without a bit of sweetness, use ¼ to ⅓ cup pear juice or another fruit juice that tastes good to you. (It's okay to be a little flexible in your post-detox life.)
- Add *plenty* of lemon or lime juice, if you like, to lighten up the

taste of your green drink. These super citrus ingredients help to alkalize the body, which in turn means fewer carb cravings. They also detoxify the liver and help flush toxins through the urinary tract. The high vitamin C content promotes healing and boosts immune system function. Talk about superfood ingredients!

- Go easy on solid ingredients if you're new to green drinks. Use a small handful of spinach leaves, versus a fistful of spinach leaves, for example. You want your drink to be light and refreshing, not sludgy and thick.
- Add cucumber (to alkalize the body and detoxify the liver) and ginger (a popular cleanse ingredient that stimulates digestion, circulation, and sweating). Both of these ingredients make for a very tasty drink!
- Start with spinach, an assortment of salad greens, and other mild green veggies if you're new to green drinks. More "hard-core" ingredients like kale, collards, and parsley tend to create a swampier-tasting drink. These superfood greens are massive health boosters (thanks to the vitamins, minerals, fiber, and high levels of anti-inflammatory and antioxidant phytochemicals they contain) and they're incredibly detoxifying, but I have to be honest with you: They don't always add up to a drink that you can appreciate right off the bat. You can always work your way up to the stronger-tasting superfood greens. Green drinks may be an acquired taste, but every drop is worth it, and, over time, you'll be surprised by how much you actually appreciate the flavor. It's all about creating a flavor profile that you can stick with.
- If you're using a blender to make your green drink, it will create some foam. Use a spatula and scrape it into the sink, if you don't care for the taste or texture. (If this is you, you're in good company: The foam makes me downright queasy.) If you're intrepid, go ahead and drink it.
- Feel free to add some extra superfood ingredients to your green drink. Try non-sweetened nut butter (for protein and fat), coconut oil (for medium-chain fatty acids—great for heart and brain

health), chia (for protein, fiber, and omega-3 fatty acids), or protein powder if you like. (For more information about superfood ingredient extras, see pages 54–57.) If you're new to cleansing, you may want to stick to the basic blueprint until you find something you like, then expand your repertoire later. Do what you'd like: I want to you to feel comfortable about experimenting with other non-sweet extras.

THE GREEN DRINK BLUEPRINTS

While you are on the 7-Day Superfood Cleanse, there are only two beverages you are required to have: water and green drinks. The green drink is enjoyed each morning with a glass of water and an optional cup of tea, as your complete breakfast, although you are encouraged to enjoy an additional green drink (or drinks) at any other time during the day, if you like. (For more information about the benefits of having a green drink for breakfast, see chapter 5.)

If you happen to be following the Everyday Cleanse Plan and really feel you need additional food with your glass of water and your green drink for breakfast, take a look at chapter 5 for solid food ideas that work with the plan. If you've chosen to follow the optional Quick Cleanse Plan on days 4 and 6 of the 7-Day Superfood Cleanse, you should to stick to water, the green drink, and optional tea. For further details about this option, take a look at chapter 5 (page 65).

BLENDER RECOMMENDATIONS

- VITAMIX (Amazon has affordable reconditioned Vitamix blenders, plus free shipping)
- BLENDTEC (I first used this brand, years ago, when I went to Natural Gourmet Cooking School, and have used it ever since. I love it even more than Vitamix. Amazon carries Blendtec and offers free shipping.)

Once you've finished the 7-Day Superfood Cleanse, you can use the *Green Drink Blueprints* if you're trying to lose some weight—or whenever you want a simple snack or a quick energy boost. It's an easy drink to pull together, using ingredients you most likely already have on hand or that are easy to find at your local supermarket. I love this green drink for breakfast—downing a large dose of veggies first thing in the morning is the best way I know to make sure my body is nourished for the day. But you really can enjoy it whenever you want—even on the road (page 55). It's a great, one-stop option for ensuring that you feel and look your best at all times. Most of the ingredients break down easily in a blender, but you'll get the best result if you use a high-power blender like a Vitamix or Blendtec. If you prefer juice to blender drinks, no problem. Instructions for the *Green Drink Juicer Blueprint* are on page 56. Ready to give your greens a whirl?

BLENDER SAFETY

If you love healthy eating, the blender is probably the most-used appliance in your kitchen. But that doesn't necessarily mean that you are using it safely. Keep these safety tips in mind before revving up your machine:

- Find a safe location for the blender, away from running water or an open flame.
- Make sure the blender cord is tucked out of the way. Make sure your machine is firmly planted on an even, level (not slanted), sturdy surface, such as a counter.
- Watch your fingers! Turn off the blender completely before adding ingredients.
- Put the lid on securely before you turn on the power—otherwise you run the risk of covering the surrounding walls and ceiling with your smoothie. Never operate your blender without the lid.

- Never operate the device if the blender jar is not securely placed on the unit.
- Regardless of how snug the lid is, hold it down while the blender is operating.
- "Pulse" is often sufficient for many blending tasks. When in doubt, start with pulsing.
- Some blenders must come to a full stop before you can safely change speed settings.
- Be careful when blending hot liquids, such as soups. The released steam can actually push the lid off while the machine is running, splattering you with scalding steam and liquids. You should fill the blender only one third to one half of its capacity, rather than filling it completely.
- When processing hot liquids, start on the lowest speed.
- Place liquid ingredients in the jar first, then add the solids.
- Cut vegetables, fruit, and other ingredients into small pieces so that they can circulate evenly around the blade.
- Avoid overworking your blender. Don't run it longer than needed, don't overload it with large and hard ingredients, and don't expect it to pulverize things that it is not capable of breaking down. If you hear a grinding noise—and certainly if you smell smoke—turn the machine off and allow it to rest for 20 minutes.
- To make cleaning easy, put a little warm water and dish detergent into the blender jar and pulse. Rinse thoroughly.
- While you can wash the blender jar and blades in the sink, never submerge the blender base in water. Your blender is an electrical appliance, and submerging it in water can produce a fatal shock. Instead, unplug it and wipe it down with a damp cloth.
- When washing the blades, be careful. They are very sharp. Rather than soaking them in soapy water (where you can accidentally cut yourself on the hidden blades), carefully wipe the blades clean with a soapy sponge or dish brush.

GREEN DRINK BLENDER BLUEPRINT
MAKES 1-2 SERVINGS

This quick, easy-to-make green drink delivers a powerful punch of antioxidants, phytonutrients, and other good stuff to keep your metabolism revving at top speed and your energy high for hours. It also works wonders on your skin, powerfully squashes cravings, and creates mental clarity.

2 cups of liquid: Water, coconut water, pure coconut milk (more caloric than coconut water), or a mixture of these. Add additional water if you want the drink to be more liquid.

1 small cucumber, or a half of an English hothouse cucumber: Peel the cucumber first, and then cut it into chunks so that your blender can handle it better. If you don't like cucumber, add a generous extra squeeze of lemon or lime juice (about a tablespoon) to keep the drink light and palatable.

The juice of 1 lemon or lime will do an excellent job of flushing toxins from the body.

1–2 small handfuls baby spinach or salad greens, such as microgreens, arugula, oak leaf lettuce, Boston leaf, mesclun mix, or anything else that strikes your fancy: Baby spinach is a particular favorite with most people because the flavors are mild, yet very tasty. Use about two small handfuls of your favorite greens for each serving. If you suffer from a health condition, please choose greens veggies that do not aggravate your condition and are sanctioned by your healthcare provider.

OPTIONAL INGREDIENTS:

4 or more leaves romaine lettuce (you can use other leafy greens if you have them around)

5–6 sprigs parsley, cilantro, dill, or other leafy herbs (with stems or without)

1 tablespoon of coconut oil, ¼ of an avocado, 2 tablespoons nut butter, or ¼ cup nuts or sunflower or pumpkin seeds—all are superb sources of brain-nourishing, cardiovascular-helping fats

1–2 tablespoons chia or hemp seed

1 teaspoon spirulina or greens powder. These will add a swampy, grassy flavor to the juice, but these powders do increase the nutrient content. Usually, I tell beginners to skip the spirulina or greens powder—you'll get plenty of nutrients without them!

½–1 scoop unflavored, vegan (non-soy, non-whey) protein powder. Do not get one of the flavored versions—they have a lot of sweetener, which will throw off your blood sugar and drain your energy.

BLENDING INSTRUCTIONS

1. Pour the chosen liquid into the blender.
2. Add all the remaining ingredients.
3. Process as long as necessary to create a smooth drink. (If your blender has options, choose the whole juice option.)
4. Skim off the foam, if you like—most people find the texture unpleasant.
5. If you're using a weaker blender, you may find it necessary to pour the liquid through a colander or strainer to remove large bits of fiber.

BLENDING GREEN DRINKS ON THE ROAD

If you have a portable blender—such as a Magic Bullet—it's a snap to stay healthy and gorgeous while you're traveling. The ingredients are the same as the *Green Drink Blender Blueprint* recipe, except:

- Opt for baby spinach or baby greens—they break down much easier in a small, portable blender. Save the heavy greens for a hardcore blender.
- For the liquid, go for water or aseptic single-serving size containers of coconut water.

GREEN DRINK JUICER BLUEPRINT

MAKES 1 SERVING

This green drink juicer blueprint has the same benefits as the blender version (page 54). I use my juicer for morning drinks and switch to my blender in the afternoon. I like the fast hit of energy I get from a fresh-pressed juice first thing in the morning, but I really need the bulk and heft of a blender drink later in the day.

1 or more small cucumbers or ½ to all of an English-style hothouse cucumber: I generally use 2 or 3 small cucumbers. Peel or don't peel the cucumber first—your choice—although if it is a non-organic cucumber (and especially if it is coated with wax), you'll want to peel it. No need to remove any seeds, though. They will go easily through the juicer. Cut the cucumber into chunks so your juicer can handle it better. If you don't like cucumber, add a generous extra measure of lemon or lime juice to keep the drink light and palatable.

1 lemon or lime (use 2 or 3 if you would like): I prefer to peel mine before juicing, since the rind can make the juice bitter.

3–4 handfuls of mature or baby spinach or salad greens: This combination of greens is a particular favorite with most people because the flavors are mild, yet very tasty. If you suffer from a health condition, please choose green veggies that do not aggravate your condition and are sanctioned by your healthcare provider.

OPTIONAL INGREDIENTS:

4 or more leaves romaine lettuce: These greens are high in calcium, copper, magnesium, manganese, phosphorous, potassium, vitamin A, vitamin B-complex, and vitamin K.

5 or more sprigs parsley, cilantro, dill, or basil (with stems, or just use the stems)

1 handful of green veggies, such as kale, Swiss chard, cabbage, celery, celery greens, beet greens, zucchini, tomatillo, or anything else that you like. Remove any tough ribs or stems.

1 or more non-green veggie, including radishes; a jalapeño or other small, not-too-spicy chile; a small carrot; a slice of jicama; a small zucchini; a few cherry tomatoes; a small handful of snow peas, snap peas, or green beans; or any other vegetable you'd like to try.

COMPLETELY OPTIONAL ADD-INS TO BE STIRRED
INTO FINISHED JUICE:

Choose one or more:

1 teaspoon spirulina or greens powder: These will add a swampy, grassy flavor to the juice, but these powders do increase the nutrient content. Usually, I tell beginners to skip the spirulina or greens powder—you'll get plenty of nutrients without them!

1 tablespoon nut butter (such as almond or cashew) or coconut oil for brain-nourishing, cardiovascular-helping fats.

1–2 tablespoons chia or hemp seed for fiber and for brain-nourishing, cardiovascular-helping fats

½–1 scoop unflavored, non-soy, non-whey protein powder. Do not get one of the flavored versions—they have a lot of sweetener, which will throw off your blood sugar and drain your energy.

JUICING INSTRUCTIONS

1. Push ingredients through the juicer.
2. If using any optional add-ins, stir them into finished juice or pour juice and add-ins into a blender and pulse to blend.

THE MASTER CLEANSE

Also known as the "Lemonade Diet," the Master Cleanse was created in 1940 by Stanley Burroughs. The program requires participants to drink water that has been boosted with lemon juice, cayenne pepper, and maple syrup for 10 or more days. Some versions strongly recommend an evening laxative. While you can lose weight on a steady diet of flavored water, it isn't the healthiest option. People who have gone on this diet have reported everything from heart palpitations to hair loss. Both times I tried it I became so dizzy I couldn't continue the cleanse.

HAVE A THYROID DISORDER?
HAVE A GREEN DRINK!

If you have a thyroid disorder, you may have been told you cannot have green drinks. Fortunately for you, this isn't true. You can absolutely and safely enjoy green drinks, as long as you avoid using ingredients that aggravate your condition. Here are safe vegetables you'll want to use, and others you'll want to avoid.

SAFE VEGGIES	VEGGIES TO USE SPARINGLY OR AVOID ALTOGETHER
Artichoke	Bok choy
Avocado	Broccoli
Beets	Broccolini
Butter leaf lettuce	Brussels sprouts
Carrot	Cabbage
Celery	Cauliflower
Chayote	Chinese broccoli
Cucumber	Collards
Green beans	Daikon
Green pepper	Kale
Herbs (cilantro, dill, parsley, etc.)	Kohlrabi
Oak lettuce (both red and green)	Millet
Okra	Mustard greens
Romaine lettuce	Peanuts
Mesclun/spring mix	Pine nuts
Micro greens	Radishes
Peas (English, snow, snap)	Red radish
Pumpkin and other winter squash	Spinach
Sea vegetables	Watercress
Tomatillo	
Zucchini and other summer squash	

OTHER DETOX-FRIENDLY DRINKS

Think of these cleansing drinks as extras—fun, tasty beverages that you can enjoy as a snack—whether you're following the Everyday Cleanse Plan or the Quick Cleanse Plan. That's right, all of these detox-friendly drinks work with both plans. The teas can also be enjoyed with breakfast or any other meal, or as a snack.

WINTER PINK DRINK: BLENDER VERSION
MAKES 1–2 SERVINGS

Full of immune system–boosting, complexion-improving phytonutrients, enzymes, vitamins, and fiber, this tart pink drink is a fun choice when you want something different. (I did mention it is tart, right?) Because it uses root vegetables, some chopping may be in order; older and weaker blenders work best with much smaller pieces than the Blendtec and Vitamix powerhouse blenders.

> ½ cup fresh or frozen cranberries or ¼–⅓ cup unsweetened cranberry juice or unsweetened tart cherry juice
> 1 small beet, chopped fine, if necessary (save the stalks and leaves to cook like chard)
> 1 small carrot, chopped fine; 1 small red pepper, chopped fine; or one small red tomato
> Juice from 1 lemon, lime, or blood orange
> 2 cups or more water or coconut water
> 1 tablespoon chia seed, optional
> 1 tablespoon coconut oil, optional
> 1 scoop protein powder, optional
> 1 handful nuts or 1 tablespoon nut butter, optional

1. Add all whole and chopped ingredients, including liquids, to a blender.
2. Purée until liquefied and smooth. Add more liquid if you'd like a thinner drink.

WINTER PINK DRINK: JUICER VERSION
MAKES 1 SERVING

The ingredients in this recipe are the same as those in the blender version on page 59. The only difference is that a juicer is used instead of a blender to make the drink. The texture, in my opinion, is nicer. But I like them both!

½ cup fresh or frozen cranberries or ¼–⅓cup unsweetened
  cranberry juice or unsweetened tart cherry juice
1 small beet chopped fine, if necessary, or ½ medium beet or
  ⅓ large beet (save the stalks and leaves to cook like chard)
1 small carrot, chopped fine; 1 small red pepper, chopped fine; or
  one small red tomato
Juice from 1 lemon, lime, or blood orange
2 cups or more water or coconut water
1 tablespoon chia seed, optional
1 tablespoon coconut oil, optional
1 scoop protein powder, optional
1 handful nuts or 1 tablespoon mild nut butter, such as cashew,
  optional

1. Run all ingredients (other than optional ingredients) through a juicer.
2. If desired, stir in as many optional ingredients as you like or pour fresh-pressed juice and optional ingredients into a blender and blend to combine.

SUMMER WATERMELON DETOX
SMOOTHIE (Use a blender)

Watermelon and its cousin, the cucumber, are considered cooling foods in many traditional healing systems (such as traditional Chinese medicine). They are said to calm irritation and frustration, as well as lower body temperature and maintain hydration—making this lovely sipper a very refreshing, cooling detox drink to enjoy when you feel warm or during hot weather.

Feel free to play with it a bit, but keep the veggies. (If you have had a particularly party-filled day, consider chopping up and adding a small, tender, inner celery rib to the mix—it's terrifically detoxifying.) I love tart flavors, so I often double the lemon or lime juice. Enjoy!

1 cup cubed red watermelon, include seeds
1 small cucumber, peeled (about 1 cup chopped)
Juice of 1 lemon or lime (about 2 tablespoons, though more is fine)
½ cup chopped romaine or other mild salad leaves
1 cup water

1. Add all ingredients to a blender and process until smooth.

SAVE THE WATERMELON RIND!

Watermelon rinds produce a wonderfully tart, detoxifying juice. If you have a juicer, simply run strips of rind through the machine, along with other veggies.

CARROT LASSI (Use a blender)
MAKES 2 SERVINGS

I use this sweet(ish) smoothie as a pick-me-up or an afternoon snack whenever I crave something creamy. You'll need a high-powered blender for this one. If you love cinnamon, cloves, or allspice, go ahead and add them!

> 1 pound carrots, peeled and finely chopped, or grated (if you have a juicer, you can use carrot pulp for this recipe)
> 2 cups unsweetened coconut milk
> 2 cups water
> ½ tablespoon coconut oil
> ½ teaspoon nutmeg
> 1 teaspoon vanilla extract or rose water, optional
> Optional: A drizzle of coconut nectar, honey, agave nectar or other sweetener to taste—if you must—although I'll be honest: Your cleanse will be deeper and more effective if you enjoy this recipe without adding a sweetener.

1. Put all ingredients in blender. Pulse until smooth and enjoy!

CITRUS ZINGER (Use a blender)
MAKES 2 SERVINGS

This recipe, a riff on cayenne-lemon water, helps detoxify the organs—and is the official drink of the Master Cleanse (page 57). I like to make a batch of this incredibly energizing drink and sip it throughout the day.

> Juice from 3 large juicy lemons or 4 limes
> ½ cup coconut water
> 1/8 teaspoon cayenne pepper
> Drizzle of coconut nectar, optional

1. Add all ingredients to a blender. Pulse until cayenne and coconut nectar are well integrated.

COCONUT COOLER (Use a blender or a cocktail shaker or any other container with a lid)
MAKES 1 SERVING

Simple and refreshing—this drink is everything a cooler should be. It's based on a recipe from my most recent book, *Coconut: The Complete Guide to the World's Most Versatile Superfood* (Sterling). It is a fantastic "mocktail" to sip when everyone around you has a glass of wine in hand.

¼ cup coconut milk (homemade or from a can, aseptic box, or refrigerated carton)
¼ cup lime juice
Coconut water ice cubes or regular ice cubes
½ cup sparkling water

1. In a cocktail shaker, Mason jar, or other type of container with a lid, shake the coconut milk and lime juice until well combined—or use a blender and pulse to blend.
2. Place one or two ice cubes in a glass and pour in the coconut milk–lime juice mixture.
3. Top off mixture with sparkling water.

LEMON WATER
MAKES 1 SERVING

I make a big glass of this every single day. I cannot imagine a day without it!

1 12-ounce glass of water, at room temperature
½ lemon

1. Squeeze lemon juice directly into the glass of water.

LEMON GINGER DETOX DRINK

This is a variation on the lemon water I drink to start my day, every day.

> 1 12-ounce glass water, at room temperature
> ½ lemon
> ½ inch knob of ginger root, peeled

1. Squeeze lemon juice directly into the glass of water.
2. Using a fine grater (such as a Microplane), grate the ginger directly into the glass of lemon water.
3. Stir and enjoy.

KEY LIME–COCONUT FRAPPÉ (Use a blender)
MAKES 2 SERVINGS

This delicious detox-friendly drink is based on a recipe in my most recent book, *Coconut: The Complete Guide to the World's Most Versatile Superfood* (Sterling). All three of my sons and I have January birthdays (the hubby's is in late December). Because each of us enjoys Key lime pie on our special day, January is dubbed Key Lime Pie Month in our household. Is it any wonder that this is one of our favorite blender drinks?

> 1 cup coconut milk (homemade or from a can, aseptic box, or
>   refrigerated carton)
> ¼ teaspoon grated lime rind
> Juice from 1 standard lime or two Key limes
> 1 tablespoon coconut oil
> ¼ cup unsweetened shredded dried coconut
> 3 ice cubes

1. Place ingredients in a blender. Process until smooth.

DETOX TEAS

Coffee is a no-no during a cleanse for a few reasons. For one, coffee causes bloating and leads to blood sugar spikes, which in turn lead to carb cravings. (Wow, is it difficult to stay on a detox menu when you're craving muffins!) In addition, research has shown that coffee raises blood pressure and increases the amount of cholesterol and other fats in the blood. On top of all that, coffee is addictive—an important detail to keep in mind as you embark on any detox program, most of which, like the 7-Day Superfood Cleanse, are designed to help break addiction to various foods!

Consequently, tea is the official hot drink of detoxers everywhere. If you are coming off a heavy coffee habit, green tea is a great substitute. Packaged green tea or green tea blends are good options, or you could enjoy the green tea drinks below.

If you can go completely without caffeine, so much the better. Caffeine is a central nervous stimulant that speeds up the heart and respiration. It forces the body to pump out cortisol, which has been linked to anxiety, and can accelerate bone loss. In addition, caffeine not only makes it difficult for the body to release toxins, it also forces the body to use a lot of energy that could be put to better use—that is, detoxifying!

Packaged detox teas (which are basically herbal teas made with one or more ingredients that speed up detoxing), as well as the straight herbal teas, can be enjoyed as often as you like. A warm cup of tea is a great pick-me-up whenever you're tempted to reach for food or coffee to relieve boredom or get a quick hit of energy.

CLASSIC LEMON-GINGER TEA

MAKES 1 SERVING

This tea, made from ingredients I always have at home, is the tea I drink most often. It is alkalizing and has detoxifying powers. It is also economical, easy to prepare, and safe to sip all day long.

1 knob ginger, peeled
1 lemon
Boiling water

1. Cut one or more slices from the knob of ginger and place it directly into a large mug.
2. Cut one or more thin slices from the lemon and place them directly into mug with the ginger.
3. Fill the mug with boiling water and allow the ginger and lemon to steep as long as you'd like. Do not sweeten.
4. Freshen with hot water and new ginger and lemon slices as desired.

STOMACH SOOTHER
MAKES 1 SERVING

If you have a sensitive digestive tract, this is a great recipe for calming a sour stomach and easing crampy large intestines. Fennel, one of the ingredients in this soother, is a time-tested remedy for flatulence, as well. Just saying . . .

> 2 teaspoons dried mint leaf (or use 2 tablespoons fresh whole leaves)
> ½ teaspoon fennel seeds

1. Add mint and fennel seeds to a large mug.
2. Fill mug with boiling water and allow to steep as long as you'd like. Do not sweeten.

THE GREEN DRINK/PROTEIN CONNECTION

Now that you've read all about the benefits of green drinks and detox teas, take a look at chapter 5, which explains how to use these cleanse-friendly beverages with the food you eat for breakfast and how to structure your mornings in order to get the biggest detox benefits from the smallest amount of effort. You'll quickly discover that adding protein to green drinks creates an alkalizing, energy-giving, nutrient-dense, detox-supportive meal that not only leaves you feeling energized, but helps you lose weight and look your best, as well.

TURMERIC TEA

MAKES 2 SERVING

Turmeric is a rhizome that is used fresh, dried, or powdered as a culinary spice. You may know it best as the ingredient that gives Indian curry its orange color. Not everyone keeps knobs of turmeric in the kitchen, but if you have easy access to the ingredient, do make this tea. Turmeric is a powerful anti-inflammatory and is known to heal the liver. The ginger, lemon, and hot pepper help boost the immune system and help the body detoxify more thoroughly.

3 cups water
1 knob ginger, peeled
1 knob fresh turmeric
1 hot pepper, such as a jalapeno or Serrano
1 lemon

1. Place water in s small saucepot over medium-low heat.
2. Cut 1 or 2 slices of ginger and add to the saucepan.
3. Cut 2 slices of turmeric and add to the saucepan.
4. Cut 2 slices of hot pepper and add to the saucepan
5. Add 2 or 3 slices of lemon to the saucepan.
6. Turn the heat to medium and allow mixture to come to a simmer.
7. Immediately turn off the heat and allow the ingredients to steep for up to 10 minutes.
8. Enjoy unsweetened.

BREAKFAST

GOOD MORNING, DETOXER! I hope you are feeling fantastic! When you start your day in a focused, healthy way, you're setting the tone for the rest of the day. Studies bear that out. The National Weight Control Registry, which tracks people who have maintained weight loss of at least 30 pounds for more than a year, has found that individuals who make healthy choices in the morning are more likely to continue making healthy choices throughout the day. Part of this is psychological—the power of a positive mindset—but part of it is also biochemical: Beginning your day with an alkalizing green juice reduces carb and sugar cravings. Without them, you'll be less tempted to have that 10 a.m. muffin and cappuccino. This is why it's essential to eat in an alkaline, detoxifying way when you're on a cleanse.

While you're detoxing, the ideal breakfast is a glass of water with lemon juice or a splash of apple cider vinegar and a green drink. If you need something hot to drink, enjoy a cup of herbal, detox, or green tea (see chapter 4). And if you absolutely need a bit more sustenance, check out the suggestions below for foods to enjoy with your glass of water and your green drink!

Regardless of whether you happen to be enjoying the Everyday Cleanse Plan or the Quick Cleanse Plan, a glass of water and a green drink will be your detox breakfast. Once the detox is over, you'll want to continue to enjoy a morning green drink, but you may want to add more food.

The *Green Drink Blender Blueprint* and the *Green Drink Juicer Blueprint*, following, are the same as the ones in chapter 4. I've repeated them here so that you don't have to flip back and forth between chapters to get the information you need when you need it.

You can also have a green drink later in the day, if you like, or any of the beverages (teas, juices, smoothies, and other beverages) in chapter 4.

GREEN DRINK BLENDER BLUEPRINT

MAKES 1–2 SERVINGS

This quick, easy-to-make green drink delivers a powerful punch of antioxidants, phytonutrients, and other good stuff to keep your energy high for hours. It also works wonders on your skin, powerfully squashes cravings, and creates mental clarity.

2 cups of liquid: Water, coconut water, pure coconut milk (more caloric than coconut water), or a mixture of these. Add additional water if you want the drink to be more liquid.

1 small cucumber, or a half of an English hothouse cucumber: Peel the cucumber first, and then cut it into chunks so that your blender can handle it better. If you don't like cucumber, add a generous extra squeeze of lemon or lime juice (about a tablespoon) to keep the drink light and palatable.

The juice of 1 lemon or lime will do an excellent job of flushing toxins from the body.

1–2 small handfuls baby spinach or salad greens, such as micro-greens, arugula, oak leaf lettuce, Boston leaf, mesclun mix, or anything else that strikes your fancy: Baby spinach is a particular favorite with most people because the flavors are mild, yet very tasty. Use about two small handfuls of your favorite greens for each serving. If you suffer from a health condition, please choose greens veggies that do not aggravate your condition and are sanctioned by your healthcare provider.

OPTIONAL INGREDIENTS:

4 or more leaves romaine lettuce (you can use other leafy greens if you have them around)

5–6 sprigs parsley, cilantro, dill, or other leafy herbs (with stems or without)

1 tablespoon of coconut oil, ¼ of an avocado, 2 tablespoons nut butter, or ¼ cup nuts or sunflower or pumpkin seeds—all are superb sources of brain-nourishing, cardiovascular-helping fats

1–2 tablespoons chia or hemp seed

1 teaspoon spirulina or greens powder. These will add a swampy, grassy flavor to the juice, but these powders do increase the nutrient content. Usually, I tell beginners to skip the spirulina or greens powder—you'll get plenty of nutrients without them!

½–1 scoop unflavored, vegan (non-soy, non-whey) protein powder. Do not get one of the flavored versions—they have a lot of sweetener, which will throw off your blood sugar and drain your energy.

BLENDING INSTRUCTIONS

1. Pour the chosen liquid into the blender.
2. Add all the remaining ingredients.
3. Process as long as necessary to create a smooth drink. (If your blender has options, choose the whole juice option.)
4. Skim off the foam, if you like—most people find the texture unpleasant.
5. If you're using a weaker blender, you may find it necessary to pour the liquid through a colander or strainer to remove large bits of fiber.

ENZYMES: WHAT ARE THEY AND WHY DO THEY MATTER?

One of the reasons I love to drink just-made green drinks is that they are filled with enzymes. These specialized protein molecules are used by our bodies for a wide range of metabolic processes, including creating and using energy, digestion, breaking down fats, building muscle, reducing inflammation, eliminating carbon dioxide from our lungs, and detoxifying the body of waste products.

Unfortunately, enzymes are not particularly hardy. They begin to lose their efficacy as soon as they are exposed to oxygen, after about 20 minutes they are no longer active. Don't worry, however, if you can't get just-pressed juice. Bottled or premade green drinks have plenty of powerful nutrients to help you get rid of excess weight, water, and toxins. In addition, the 7-Day Superfood Cleanse menu is rich in enzymes, so if you don't get them in your drink, I promise that you are getting them elsewhere.

GREEN DRINK JUICER BLUEPRINT
MAKES 1 SERVING

This green drink juicer blueprint has the same benefits as the blender version (page 70). I use my juicer for morning drinks and switch to my blender in the afternoon. I like the fast hit of energy I get from a fresh-pressed juice first thing in the morning, but I really need the bulk and heft of a blender drink later in the day.

1 or more small cucumbers or ½ to all of an English-style hothouse cucumber: I generally use 2 or 3 small cucumbers. Peel or don't peel the cucumber first—your choice—although if it is a non-organic cucumber (and especially if it is coated with wax), you'll want to peel it. No need to remove any seeds, though. They will go easily through the juicer. Cut the cucumber into chunks so your juicer can handle it better. If you don't like cucumber, add a generous extra measure of lemon or lime juice to keep the drink light and palatable.

1 lemon or lime (use 2 or 3 if you would like): I prefer to peel mine before juicing, since the rind can make the juice bitter.

3–4 handfuls of mature or baby spinach or salad greens: This combination of greens is a particular favorite with most people because the flavors are mild, yet very tasty. If you suffer from a health condition, please choose green veggies that do not aggravate your condition and are sanctioned by your healthcare provider.

OPTIONAL INGREDIENTS:

4 or more leaves romaine lettuce: These greens are high in calcium, copper, magnesium, manganese, phosphorous, potassium, vitamin A, vitamin B-complex, and vitamin K.

5 or more sprigs parsley, cilantro, dill, or basil (with stems, or just use the stems)

1 handful of green veggies, such as kale, Swiss chard, cabbage, celery, celery greens, beet greens, zucchini, tomatillo, or anything else that you like. Remove any tough ribs or stems.

1 or more non-green veggie, including radishes; a jalapeño or other small, not-too-spicy chile; a small carrot; a slice of jicama; a small zucchini; a few cherry tomatoes; a small handful of snow peas, snap peas, or green beans; or any other vegetable you'd like to try.

COMPLETELY OPTIONAL ADD-INS TO BE STIRRED
INTO FINISHED JUICE

Choose one or more:

1 teaspoon spirulina or greens powder: These will add a swampy, grassy flavor to the juice, but these powders do increase the nutrient content. Usually, I tell beginners to skip the spirulina or greens powder—you'll get plenty of nutrients without them!

1 tablespoon nut butter (such as almond or cashew) or coconut oil for brain-nourishing, cardiovascular-helping fats.

1–2 tablespoons chia or hemp seed for fiber and for brain-nourishing, cardiovascular-helping fats

½–1 scoop unflavored, non-soy, non-whey protein powder. Do not get one of the flavored versions—they have a lot of sweetener, which will throw off your blood sugar and drain your energy.

JUICING INSTRUCTIONS

1. Push ingredients through the juicer.
2. If using any optional add-ins, stir them into finished juice or pour juice and add-ins into a blender and pulse to blend.

WHAT IF YOU NEED MORE FOOD?

If you are still hungry after you've had your green drink, add a bit of fat (maybe a tablespoon of coconut oil or a sliver of avocado) and some protein (for example, protein powder or nut butter) to your next drink, or snack on ¼ cup of nuts or seeds, or a cup of canned or home-cooked beans (try stirring in a tablespoon or more of salsa or chopped veggies to warm things up) or a cup of any of the bean, grain, veggie, salad, or soup recipes in the lunch or dinner chapters in this book. The addition of protein and fat will help keep you satisfied longer, so you won't be tempted to turn to bagels, muffins, and breakfast pastries.

WHAT IF I CAN'T MAKE MY OWN GREEN DRINK FOR BREAKFAST?

Sometimes making your own green drink for breakfast is impossible. Whether you don't have enough time in the morning to devote to your green drink or you are traveling, you do have other options. They may not be quite as fabulous as a just-made green drink, but they are pretty good backups nonetheless! Try some of these:

- Have a green salad for breakfast. That's right. Go ahead and make a green salad—or pick one up from a salad bar or restaurant. It doesn't matter what greens are in the salad as long as you stick with a vinaigrette or nut-based salad dressing. Add a handful of nuts or beans if you want a bit of protein, but avoid dairy products (cheese or creamy dressings), animal protein, and wheat products. Avoid dried and fresh fruit, too.

- Help yourself to a low-sugar, no-fruit, premade bottled green drink. Once upon a time the only bottled green juice you could get was at health food stores. My how things have changed! Today, you can even by green juice in coffee houses! However, just because you can buy these yummy drinks everywhere, doesn't mean they are all good for you. I hate to be the bearer of bad news, but the majority of pre-bottled green drinks go heavy on banana purée, apple juice, and other fruity ingredients that contribute outrageous amounts of sugars (some in the 23–34 gram range). Also, when you mix sweet fruits and veggies in a juice, you can become crampy and gassy—plus, all that fruit sugar does wacky things to your blood sugar levels and can create cravings, fatigue, and irritability. Many brands of bottled green juices—such as Odwalla and Naked—are almost all banana purée or grape or apple juice with a smidgen of spinach for color. You do not want that. Instead, you want something powerful, detoxifying, and alkalizing to keep your energy high. My favorite nationally available green drinks include:

  - **Evolution Juice** (www.evolutionfresh.com): Try the Essential Greens; Essential Greens with Lime; Coconut Water and

Greens; Smooth Greens; or Organic Avocado Greens (which has more of a smoothie consistency). You can get these in many supermarkets and at Starbucks (since the brand is manufactured by Starbucks's parent company.)

- **Suja** (www.sujajuice.com): This brand is available in Whole Foods and many supermarkets. These green drinks are a little higher in sugar than the Evolution juices but are still only 14 grams or less, so they should be fine for you. Choose Green Essentials (it has the least amount of sugar and can be a little bitter), Fiji, Glow, or Power Greens.
- **Juice Press** (www.juicepress.com/cold-pressed-juice): You can find these juices in some grocery stores, or order them directly from the website and have them delivered to your home or office. Some of their juices contain huge amounts of sugar, however, so stick to Mother Earth, Gravity, The Meal, Anti-Aging, Simple Green, Doctor Earth, or OMG!

- Enjoy a fresh-pressed juice from a health food store or juice joint. This is my favorite option because the juice is made in front of your eyes and if you drink it within 20 minutes or so of pressing, you'll get powerful, immune-system boosting enzymes as bonus! And you can ask the person who's preparing the drink to customize the drink according to your taste and health needs.

6

LUNCH

WHEN YOU'RE ON A CLEANSE, WHAT you eat for lunch becomes essential. It can make or break your body's ability to detox.

I say this not to scare you, but because most of us don't give too much thought to lunch. We bring something from home—maybe the same thing every single day—or we run out to the corner deli or takeout shop. We may even chow on fast food—or skip lunch altogether. The point is, most of us see lunch as, well, any old thing to help get us through the rest of the day, and although that may be true on a certain level, the fact is that our bodies actually have very specific requirements at midday. In fact, if you don't eat the right foods, you may feel tired, cold, spacey, and apathetic, or you may experience digestive issues, mood swings, and anxiety. To avoid all that misery and gain the energy you need, in order to maintain focus and mental acuity, and to enjoy a stable, happy mood, you need protein, fat, vitamins, minerals, fiber, and phytonutrients to help keep your immune system strong, your nervous system soothed, and your metabolism running on high. The right foods will alkalize your body and prevent those afternoon cravings for coffee, carbs, and sweets.

In short, the ideal detox lunch consists of protein, greens (and other bright-colored veggies), plus good old H_2O. The meals in this chapter will offer you everything you need to maintain your cleanse while supporting your health. They'll leave you feeling light and energetic and won't cause afternoon cravings. Choose what you love, or (for those of you who don't want to cook) look at my suggestions for safe takeout options.

All of the recipes in this chapter are appropriate for both the Everyday Cleanse Plan and the optional Quick Cleanse Plan. (If you are following the Quick Cleanse Plan on days 4 and 6 of the 7-Day Superfood Cleanse, lunch will be the only solid food meal of the day—breakfast, snacks, and dinner will be liquid.)

COMPLETE MEAL OPTIONS

A combination of protein and veggies, the recipes for complete meals in this chapter, make it easy to whip up delicious, one-dish detox lunches. Enjoy one of them—or a similar takeout meal for lunch—and you don't need anything else. Having said that, feel free to add a cup of veggie-based (no dairy and no wheat) soup or a small side salad or side serving of veggies, if you'd like more food. The *Grain or Bean Salad Blueprint*, (page 80), is much more flexible than a traditional salad recipe because it allows you to swap in ingredients you like and happen to have on hand. You don't have to rush out and buy anything special (or that you wouldn't normally eat) to make the blueprint work for you, and it includes hearty ingredients that will satisfy your appetite and keep your energy high. Just be sure to not to use any ingredients that you don't digest well or that your healthcare practitioner has advised you to avoid.

TOXINS TO AVOID
IN YOUR LUNCHBOX

For years I packed lunches in a collection of cleaned-up takeout containers, plastic sandwich bags, and aluminum foil. These were cheap and easy to find, and they did the job. They also exposed me to BPA (bisphenol A), PVC (polyvinyl chloride), phthalates (chemicals used to soften vinyl), aluminum, and lead, none of which was good for my health, my weight, or my body's natural ability to detoxify. Here's a rundown of these substances and how they affect your health:

• BPA (BISPHENOL A). BPA is an industrial chemical that has been used to make certain plastics (such as plastic bottles, including water bottles, and the lining of food cans) since the 1960s. Exposure to BPA can affect the brain, behavior, and prostate gland of fetuses, infants, and children. If a plastic product is not labeled, take a look at its recycle code. Plastics marked with recycle codes 3 or 7 may be made with BPA.

• PVC (POLYVINYL CHLORIDE). This popular thermoplastic is cheap, lightweight, and malleable, making it a popular additive in plastic bottles (including water bottles), cups, and some food storage containers (hopefully none you are using to carry your lunches in!). PVC is often referred to as the "poison plastic" because of the toxins it can release when it is exposed to heat or decomposes in landfills. PVC has been linked to cancer, birth defects, endocrine disruption, asthma, and lung problems.

• PHTHALATES. This class of chemicals is used to soften vinyl so that it can be molded, and causes a wide range of adverse health problems, including liver, kidney, and lung damage, as well as reproductive system and sexual development abnormalities. You are most likely to come in contact with phthalates in soft lunch bags and totes. The Environmental Protection Agency has listed phtlates as a "probable human carcinogen, based on studies that have shown an increased rate of cancers in rats and mice that were exposed to phtlates, as opposed to a control group of rats and mice that were not exposed to phthalates."

• ALUMINUM. There are mixed reports on the safety of aluminum foil. Some food safety experts do not see a safety issue, while others believe that aluminum leaches into food. High levels of aluminum exposure have been correlated with neurological declines in balance, coordination, and memory, as well as reproductive toxicity.

• LEAD. Lead is sometimes added to vinyl as a stabilizer, helping vinyl bend, then bounce back to its original shape. It's also cheap and easy to use, which makes it a favorite ingredient in the making of vinyl lunch bags, boxes, and totes. Unfortunately, lead is a neurotoxin that, at low levels, can impair cognitive function. It is particularly harmful to young children's developing brains and nervous systems. Unfortunately, you can't always know which lunch boxes do and don't contain lead. The nonprofit Center for Environmental Health, based in Oakland, California, tested lunch boxes in 2005 and found that 25 percent contained lead.

GRAIN OR BEAN SALAD BLUEPRINT
MAKES 2 SERVINGS

Everyone needs a great, easy, flexible blueprint for a yummy, healthful, high-protein salad—a hearty, fiber-filled dish made with high-protein beans, lentils, dried peas, and/or superfood grains such as millet, amaranth, quinoa, teff, buckwheat, barley, black rice, or another whole-grain rice.

The *Grain or Bean Salad Blueprint* is fun to make, easy to customize, and super portable—perfect for bringing to the office for lunch or on a picnic). It is designed to deliver the nutrients your body needs to help keep your energy high all day.

Don't forget to sprinkle in a liberal amount of your favorite herbs (which are superfoods, by the way, thanks to their ultra-high phytonutrient content), along with a bunch of chopped veggies and your favorite spices—superfood ingredients that are loaded with anti-inflammatory nutrients. Grab your favorite vinegar and oil, and voilà, you have a fabulous salad that you can't wait to enjoy. Is it lunchtime yet?

¼ cup (or more) vinaigrette or your favorite salad dressing
  (homemade or store-bought)
1 tablespoon (or more) of your favorite herb or mix of herbs
1 garlic clove, minced
¼ cup onion, scallions, or shallots
Pinch salt and pepper
4 cups cooked beans or grain of your choice
1 cup chopped cooked or raw vegetables
1 cup plant protein of your choice (optional; you can use animal
  protein when you are not on a cleanse)
¼ cup (or more) nuts or seeds, for crunch (optional)

1. In a large bowl, whisk together the salad dressing, herbs, garlic, onion, salt, and pepper.
2. Add in all the other ingredients, stirring gently until well coated.
3. Adjust salt and pepper.
4. While you can eat this right away, it will taste so much livelier if you allow to sit for 30 minutes or more so flavors can blend.

QUINOA SUPERFOOD SALAD

MAKES 2 3-CUP SERVINGS

This is a lovely, bright-tasting pilaf/salad hybrid. It is loaded with detoxifying cilantro and cucumber and filled with superfoods, including pomegranate seeds (fiber, vitamins C and E), chickpeas (molybdenum, manganese, folate, fiber, protein), quinoa (anti-inflammatory phytonutrients, fiber, protein), and avocado (pantothenic acid, oleic acid, fiber, glutathione, vitamin K).

DRESSING

½ cup freshly squeezed orange juice
3 tablespoons freshly squeezed lemon or lime juice (or a
   combination)
1 teaspoon raw honey, coconut nectar, or agave (optional)
3 tablespoons extra-virgin olive oil or coconut oil
1 or 2 cloves minced garlic
½ heaping teaspoon salt, or to taste
Pinch black pepper, or to taste

SALAD

1 medium cucumber, peeled, seeded, and diced
½ cup medium red onion, minced
¼ cup fresh minced cilantro (or a combination of parsley and
   cilantro)
1 cup pomegranate seeds
3 cups cooked quinoa
2 cups cooked or 1 15-ounce can chickpeas, well-drained
1 avocado, cut into small cubes
Salt and freshly ground black pepper

1. In a small bowl, whisk together the dressing ingredients. Set aside.
2. In a large bowl or food storage container, combine the cucumber, onion, cilantro, and pomegranate seeds. Stir gently to combine.
3. Add the quinoa and toss gently.
4. Add the chickpeas and avocado and toss gently.
5. Drizzle the dressing over the mixture. Toss gently to combine. Add salt and pepper to taste.

GINGERED MILLET WITH JAPANESE VEGGIES

MAKES 2 3-CUP SERVINGS

Millet is another one of my favorite superfoods. This ancient grain nourished centuries of Africans, Indians, Asians, and Europeans. Millet boasts protein and fiber, as well as large amounts of magnesium, iron, calcium, phosphorus, and potassium. It also contains B-complex vitamins, vitamin E, and amino acids. Here, millet is paired with the superfood, coconut, along with members of the cruciferous family, beans, and sunflower seeds.

1 cup millet
2–3 tablespoons minced fresh ginger
½ teaspoon sea salt
3 cups water or vegetable broth
3 tablespoons sesame oil (you can use extra virgin olive oil or
    coconut oil if you don't have sesame oil—though sesame oil
    tastes fantastic in this recipe!)
3 tablespoons coconut vinegar or apple cider vinegar
4 cups cooked or 2 15-ounce cans black beans, drained and rinsed
2 tablespoons coconut oil
1 carrot, finely diced
3 radishes, finely diced
½ cup snow peas or sugar snap peas, chopped
½ cup shredded red cabbage
3 scallions, thinly sliced
Salt and freshly ground black pepper, to taste
¼ cup sunflower seeds or walnuts or another seed or nut

1. Place the millet and the ginger in a small saucepan. Add ½ teaspoon of salt and water or broth. Bring to a boil, stir once, then reduce heat and simmer, covered, for 25 minutes.

2. As the millet cooks, whisk together the sesame oil, vinegar, and salt in a large bowl. Set aside.

3. Check the millet. When it is done, remove from the heat and allow to rest for 10 minutes.

4. Fluff with a fork and add the beans. Set aside.

5. Warm the coconut oil in a large sauté pan. Flash-sauté* the carrot,

radishes, snow peas, cabbage, and scallions until firm-tender. Season with salt and pepper.

6. Scrape the sautéed veggies into the bowl with the vinaigrette and stir to coat.

7. Stir in the millet-bean mixture and sunflower seeds and stir again, to coat.

*Flash-sauté: The word *sauté* is French for *jumped* or *bounced*. I'll bet you've sautéed something, even if you didn't realize it! To sauté, simply heat some oil in a pan, add food, and quickly jiggle or stir the food in the pan so that it is thoroughly coated in oil and cooked to a crisp-tender state. Flash-sautéing is just another fancy term for a very quick way to cook the food in only 3–5 minutes. It's a great method for barely tenderizing food while keeping its texture intact and helping to meld flavors into a cohesive blend.

BLACK-EYED PEA SALAD
MAKES: 2 3-CUP SERVINGS

I love black-eyed pea salads, often known as Texas caviar. I serve them as a dip or salsa at parties and eat them as a salad. This dish will give you protein, fiber, vitamins, and minerals!

DRESSING
Juice of 1 lemon
2 tablespoons apple cider vinegar
2 tablespoons whole grain mustard
Salt and pepper to taste
¼ cup extra virgin olive oil

SALAD
4 cups cooked or 2 15-ounce cans black-eyed peas well-drained
2 cups of your favorite raw veggies, cut into a small dice
¼ cup minced fresh cilantro, parsley, chives, dill, or a
    combination of these herbs

1. In a bowl, whisk together the dressing ingredients to combine.

2. In a large bowl, combine the beans, veggies, and herbs.

3. Pour the dressing over the salad and mix well. For the best flavor, allow the salad to sit for an hour or more before eating.

MEXICALI QUINOA PILAF

Every ingredient in this one-dish meal contributes a large number of nutrients, making this your next go-to meal. Take it to work and you will feel energized and alert. Feel free to play around with the recipe—add a cup of chopped leftover veggies, use a different type of legume or herb, and so on.

    2 tablespoons coconut oil
    1 cup diced red, orange, or yellow bell pepper
    1 cup zucchini, chayote, or summer squash, diced
    2 garlic cloves, minced
    3 or more scallions, chopped
    ¼ teaspoon cayenne powder
    ¼ teaspoon chili powder
    1 cup canned coconut milk (preferably full fat)
    2 cups cooked or canned black beans (about 1 15-ounce can),
        rinsed and drained
    3 cups cooked quinoa
    ¼ teaspoon salt
    ½ cup chopped pepitas (pumpkin seeds) or sunflower seeds
    ¼ cup chopped cilantro

1. Add the coconut oil to a large skillet over medium heat and sauté the peppers, squash, garlic, scallions, cayenne powder, and chili powder. Sauté until just tender, about 5 minutes.
2. Add the coconut milk and black beans to the veggie mixture, cover the skillet, and cook for 5 minutes over medium heat.
3. Stir in the quinoa and salt and allow to sit until cool.
4. Garnish with the pepitas and cilantro and serve.

WHAT ARE ANTHOCYANINS?

Anthocyanins, antioxidants found in black rice, have been found to help fight heart disease, diabetes, and Alzheimer's disease. They are being studied for their role in helping fight cancer.

BLACK RICE SALAD
MAKES 2 3-CUP SERVINGS

Black rice has a lovely nutty taste and toothsome bite that I find addictive. This recipe features a host of ingredients rich in antioxidants, fiber, and protein. You'll love it!

DRESSING
3 tablespoons lemon juice
2 tablespoons white wine vinegar
2 teaspoons coconut syrup (nectar), honey, or brown rice syrup
¼ cup extra-virgin olive oil
Salt and pepper, to taste

SALAD
1½ cups uncooked black rice
2½ cups lightly salted water
Salt and pepper, to taste
½ cup walnuts
5 scallions, thinly sliced
2 cups frozen lima beans, thawed
1 cup grape tomatoes, halved
1 cup snow or snap peas, thinly sliced
Salt and pepper, to taste

1. Whisk the lemon juice, vinegar, and coconut nectar in a small bowl. Whisking constantly, gradually drizzle in the oil. Season with salt and pepper to taste.
2. Cook the rice in a medium saucepan of boiling salted water until tender, 35–40 minutes. Drain well and set aside to cool.
3. In a large bowl, toss the walnuts, scallions, lima beans, tomatoes, and snow peas together with the dressing.
4. Add the cooled rice and toss again. Season with salt and pepper to taste.

GRAINS: ENJOY WITH A VEGGIE (OR TWO)

I love stir-fries, ragouts, curries . . . and I'm wild about sauced veggies eaten over grains. It's a good thing these make such great detox
lunches! If grain-and-veggie combos call to you, as well, choose one
of the recipes below, which feature high-protein superfood grains like
millet and quinoa, and pair it with one or two veggies. Just remember:
no dairy, soy, or wheat!

BROWN RICE MEDLEY
2 1½-CUP SERVINGS

This is a lovely brown rice salad. Add more veggies, if you like, or even
some legumes. The herbal-rich vinaigrette helps the body detoxify and
is super delicious.

> 1 cup (packed) chopped fresh chives, or a combination of chives,
>   dill, parsley, and/or cilantro
> ½ cup plus 2 tablespoons extra-virgin olive oil
> 2 tablespoons fresh lemon juice, plus more for seasoning, if
>   desired
> 1 teaspoon kosher salt
> 1½ cups summer squash, such as zucchini, lightly squeezed
>   to remove liquid
> 2 cups cooked brown rice
> 2 scallions, thinly sliced
> ½ cup toasted salted sunflower seeds, pepitas, or chopped
>   almonds
> Salt and black pepper

1. Purée the chives, oil, lemon juice, and 1 teaspoon of kosher salt in
a food processor until smooth. Strain the chive vinaigrette through a
fine-mesh sieve into a small bowl.
2. In a large bowl, toss together the summer squash, rice, scallions,
seeds, and herb vinaigrette. Season to taste with salt, pepper, and more
lemon juice, if desired.

MILLET WITH ROASTED SUNFLOWER SEEDS

MAKES 3 1½-CUP SERVINGS

Millet is a gluten-free seed that we use as a culinary grain. It is high in protein, calcium, and other minerals.

1 cup sunflower seeds
2¼ cups water
1 cup millet
Pinch of sea salt

1. Dry-roast the sunflower seeds in a skillet over medium heat until they release a nutty aroma, approximately 4 minutes.
2. Bring the water to a boil and add the millet and seeds.
3. Cover and simmer for 30 minutes.
4. When the millet is done, fluff and let sit for 10 minutes.
5. Season with salt and enjoy with the veggie sides in this chapter.

NON-TOXIC WAYS TO PACK YOUR LUNCH

Because you've chosen to dive in and clean up your eating habits, I am going to ask you to clean up your food containers by choosing toxin-free wrapping, bags, and containers. Here's a handy list of options:
- STAINLESS STEEL LUNCH CONTAINERS, including Bento Duo by LunchBots, 3-Tier Tiffin by Life Without Plastic, and various-sized food canisters by Klean Kanteen
- GLASS CONTAINERS, such as square glass Meal Cube or Lunch Bowl by Wean Green
- SAFE FOOD WRAP, such as Organic Cotton Sandwich Wrap by Eco Lunch Gear or Food Kozy Clear by U-Konserve
- BROWN PAPER LUNCH BAGS, the old-fashioned kind that you can buy at grocery stores everywhere
- CLOTH FOOD BAGS, including LunchSkins Reusable Snack Bag
- BIODEGRADABLE FOOD BAGS, such as Compostable Sandwich Bags by BioBag

TRY NOT TO EAT AT YOUR DESK

You may have heard the recent hoopla about eating at your desk. Several news outlets reported a host of detractions and ills that come with in-office eating, among them:

- BACTERIA AND OTHER MICROBES. A team of researchers from the University of Arizona measured the bacterial count on several office surfaces. What they found will amaze you: Your desk and keyboard contain 10 billion bacteria, more than four hundred times more than an average toilet seat. Is that where you want to eat?

- MINDLESS EATING AND OVEREATING. I know I talk a lot about mindful eating, but that's only because it is an important way to allow your body to feel full so you avoid overstuffing yourself. Eating too much food at a time hampers detoxing. When you eat at your desk, your focus is on your work, your email, or your Facebook page, instead of what you are eating or how quickly you are eating it. You may be so engrossed in web surfing that you finish your food without realizing that you've eaten it, then, feeling cheated, you may be tempted to find more food so that you can fully experience the satisfaction of eating.

- INEFFICIENT DIGESTION AND NUTRIENT METABOLISM. Your body gets ready to digest food by secreting saliva in your mouth and gastric juices in your stomach. If you are paying attention to something other than your food, your body doesn't secrete the amount of saliva or gastric juices required to thoroughly digest food. This means that if you are not digesting well, you aren't getting the nutrients you need to detox and power-up your body to function at top rev. And you may even experience digestive discomfort, such as bloating, indigestion, heartburn, gas, and constipation.

- LESS PRODUCTIVITY. Getting up and moving to the cafeteria, break room, or park in order to eat your lunch is great for detoxification. It increases circulation and allows healing and energizing oxygen to reach and refresh all parts of your body, including your brain, which boosts job productivity, along with body functions that include detoxification.

- HABITUAL EATING. Eating at your desk every day creates a deeply ingrained habit that causes your brain to associate your workspace with food. Once that habit is cemented, you will always want snacks when you sit down to work, whether or not your body is actually hungry. This leads to overeating, which in turn makes it difficult for your body to detoxify.

COCONUT BROWN RICE

MAKES 6 SERVINGS

This is a very basic recipe—and a very good one. Coconut rice is one of my kids' favorite side dishes. Full of fiber, protein, and an incredible array of minerals (manganese, selenium, magnesium), this dish is the perfect foil for curries, sautés, stir-fries, and other saucy dishes. It's also a great base for more elaborate combos: Add nuts, dried fruits, beans, and so on, and you have a pilaf.

2½ cups water
1 can coconut milk
½ teaspoon salt
2 cups brown rice

1. In a medium saucepan, bring the water, coconut milk, and salt to a boil.
2. Add the rice, stir just once, reduce the heat to low, and cover.
3. Simmer for about 45 minutes (without stirring even once—that's what makes rice mushy!) or until rice is cooked and grains are separate and fluffy, with no liquid left in the pot. You can lift the lid once or twice while rice cooks to check on it, but quickly replace the lid.

COCONUT QUINOA
MAKES 2 SERVINGS

You have probably heard of the superseed quinoa. This tiny seed—which we treat as a culinary grain—is a complete protein, which means it contains all the amino acids a body needs to efficiently metabolize the food's protein. And wow, does quinoa contain a lot of protein: 24 grams per 1 cup serving! Quinoa also contains generous amounts of fiber, magnesium, manganese, iron, vitamins B2 and B6, lysine, and phytochemicals that help the brain, heart, and immune system. This delicious dish pairs quinoa with coconut—another versatile superfood—resulting in a delectable, portable, nourishing midday nosh.

1 tablespoon liquid coconut oil
⅓ cup finely diced carrot
⅓ cup diced celery
¼ cup diced onion
1 garlic clove, minced
1 teaspoon grated fresh ginger
4 cups cooked quinoa
3 tablespoons unsweetened shredded dried coconut
½ tablespoon lime juice
Cilantro for garnish, optional

1. Warm the coconut oil a large sauté pan over medium heat. Add the carrot, celery, and onion, and sauté until tender.
2. Add the garlic and ginger and cook for just about a minute more.
3. Remove from heat and stir in the quinoa, shredded coconut, and lime juice, and garnish with cilantro.

VEGGIES: ENJOY ONE OR TWO OF THESE WITH A GRAIN

Other than salad, I find that many of my clients don't eat a lot of veggies for lunch. This saddens me! Vegetables should be a foundation of your diet—certainly while you're on the 7-Day Superfood Cleanse, but also afterward, when you've gone back to "real-life" eating. So, in the hope of luring you into trying something that perhaps is new to you, I'm eager to offer you some of my favorite superfood-based, detox-friendly vegetable recipes, all of which are ideal for lunch. But you can also use them as dinner side dishes or snacks—or even have them with breakfast, if you like. All of the recipes are loaded with nutrient-dense power foods, such as nuts, seeds, beans, cruciferous veggies, coconut, leafy greens, deeply colored root veggies, and so forth. If you don't like to cook, feel free to hit a healthy takeout place or a prepared food bar (like the ones you find in Whole Foods Market and many other health food stores) and purchase something comparable. Your body will thank you with all-day energy, focus, mental acuity, and the welcome absence of crazy carb cravings! The right foods at lunch make an enormous difference to the kind of afternoon and evening you'll have.

SIDE SALAD BLUEPRINT

MAKES 2 1½-CUP SERVINGS

It wasn't until after I began writing recipes that I learned that people actually follow recipes for salads. I had always viewed salads as an infinitely variable dish, based on whatever happened to be on hand—some greens, maybe some leftovers from the previous meal, canned beans, nuts, dried or fresh herbs, and so on, and a dressing that could be thrown together quickly. If you are someone who likes to follow recipes, here you go. . . but don't forget to experiment with the ingredients!

DRESSING

2 tablespoons coconut vinegar, or any other type of vinegar you enjoy

2 tablespoons coconut aminos (leave out if you'd like, but coconut aminos are helpful detoxifying agents and add a wonderful savory taste to dressings and other foods)

1 to 2 tablespoon liquid coconut oil, or another oil, such as extra virgin olive oil

1 teaspoon coconut sugar or another natural sweetener, such as maple syrup, optional

½ to 1 teaspoon mustard of choice, optional

Salt and pepper to taste

SALAD

3 cups salad greens of choice

½ cup chopped vegetable or a mix of vegetables of choice, optional

¼ cup chopped fresh herbs, optional

1. In a large bowl, whisk together the coconut vinegar, coconut aminos, coconut oil, coconut sugar, and mustard, if using, and salt and pepper.

2. To the bowl, add the salad greens and optional ingredients. Toss until all the ingredients are coated with dressing. Serve immediately.

TAKE-TO-WORK INSTRUCTIONS: Place all the veggies in a food container. Make the dressing ahead of time and put it in a separate small container. When you're ready to eat, drizzle the dressing onto the salad and shake the salad to distribute dressing.

BRAISED COCONUT SPINACH AND CHICKPEAS WITH LEMON

MAKES 2 1½-CUP SERVINGS

Tender braised greens and chickpeas create a beautiful ragout-like dish that is lovely served over brown rice, millet, quinoa, polenta, potatoes, mashed cauliflower, puréed sweet potatoes, or anything else you like. Your taste buds will thank you. So will your body: This dish is high in vitamins A, C, and E; protein; zinc; magnesium; fiber; and more.

2 tablespoons liquid coconut oil
1 small yellow onion, diced
5–6 garlic cloves, minced
1 tablespoon grated fresh ginger
¼ to ½ teaspoon red pepper flakes
1 15-ounce can chickpeas, drained
1 pound baby spinach
1 15-ounce can coconut milk
2 tablespoons lemon juice
¼ cup tomato paste
Salt and pepper to taste

1. Heat the coconut oil in a large saucepan over medium-high heat. Add the onion and cook for about 5 minutes or until it begins to brown.

2. Add the garlic, ginger, and red pepper. Cook for 3 minutes, stirring frequently.

3. Add the chickpeas and cook over high heat for about 2 minutes or until the chickpeas begin to turn golden.

4. Add the spinach, working in batches as spinach wilts, to fit all spinach into pan.

5. Add the coconut milk, lemon juice, tomato paste, salt, and pepper. Bring to a simmer, then turn down the heat and cook for 10 minutes, or until the chickpeas are warmed through.

6. Adjust salt and pepper before serving.

ROASTED VEGGIES IN COCONUT OIL

MAKES 4 1-CUP SERVINGS

Everyone needs a good roasted veggie recipe. If you don't believe me, just try this one and you'll know what I mean. I make at least one pan of roasted veggies a week, varying the veggies each time, according to what I have around. The finished dish is often eaten straight from the baking pan, sprinkled into pilafs and salads, or as an after-school snack. Play with this recipe—you can use equal amounts of other veggies, such as radishes, rutabaga, fennel, burdock, kohlrabi, broccoli stems, brussels sprouts, or any other vegetable that strikes your fancy! You can even roast all sweet potatoes, all beets, or whatever you like.

4–5 carrots, peeled
2 medium onions, peeled
1 acorn squash, cleaned and peeled
1 large sweet potato, peeled
3–4 small red potatoes
1 medium red beet, peeled
¼ cup coconut oil or extra virgin olive oil
Salt and pepper to taste
1 or more tablespoons fresh chopped herb, such as thyme, optional

1. Preheat oven to 425°F.
2. Cut all the vegetables into similarly-sized pieces.
3. Place the vegetables in a bowl. Drizzle them with coconut oil and sprinkle with salt and pepper and the optional herb. Using clean hands, toss the veggies until all are coated.
4. Place the vegetables in a single layer on one or two rimless baking sheets.
5. Roast for 25–35 minutes, or until all the vegetables are tender, turning them once.
6. Adjust the salt and pepper.

CLASSIC GREENS
MAKES 2 1½-CUP SERVINGS

You can use collards, mustard greens, kohlrabi leaves, cabbage, turnip greens, or another green in this recipe, as well. Play around with it!

1 bunch kale
2 tablespoons olive oil
½ tablespoon fresh ginger, minced
1 clove garlic, minced
Salt and pepper to taste
1 medium-size yellow onion, diced

1. Wash the kale, cut away the stems and tough inside ribs (save them for the juicer). Cut or tear the leaves into small pieces.
2. Add the oil to a sauté pan and warm over medium heat.
3. Add the ginger, garlic, and salt to taste. Sauté for one minute.
4. Add the onion and sauté for a few more minutes.
5. Add the kale, stir well, and then add a splash of water. Cover and allow to cook for 8–10 minutes.
6. Check for desired tenderness and adjust the salt and pepper.

INDIAN GREENS

MAKES 2 1½-CUP SERVINGS

My clients makes fun of me because I am obsessed with cumin. This is one of my favorite, fast, "cuminified" ways to make greens. The recipe calls for Swiss chard (silver beet, for my UK and Aussie friends), but if you don't like chard or can't eat it because of a health concern, substitute any other green. You may have to adjust the cooking time and add a bit of water, but all will be delicious (and detoxifying) in the end.

1 bunch Swiss chard
2 tablespoons coconut oil
1 teaspoon black mustard seeds
1 teaspoon ground cumin
1 teaspoon ground coriander
½ teaspoon sea salt
Salt and pepper to taste
¼ cup canned coconut milk

1. Wash the chard, cut out the stems (save for another use or to juice), and chop the leaves into 1-inch pieces.

2. Heat the oil in a frying pan over medium-high heat.

3. When the oil is hot, add the mustard seeds and cook, stirring for 1 minute.

4. Add the cumin and coriander, and cook for another 30 seconds, stirring.

5. Add the chard and salt. Mix well and cook 3–5 minutes, until the chard is wilted.

6. Turn off the heat, stir in the coconut milk, and adjust the salt and pepper.

SAUTÉED BROCCOLI RABE

MAKES 2 1½-CUP SERVINGS

I was an adult before I got around to trying broccoli rabe, and wow, was I hooked! I am attracted to bitter foods, which explains my affection for this nutritious Italian green. It happens to contain vitamins A, C, and K; lutein; potassium; iron; calcium; and fiber. This recipe works well for regular broccoli, as well.

    1 bunch broccoli rabe
    2 tablespoons olive oil
    2 cloves garlic, minced
    Salt and pepper to taste
    2 tablespoons water

1. Wash the broccoli rabe and cut the stems into 1–2 inch pieces.
2. Warm the oil in a pan and add the garlic. Sauté for a few minutes.
3. Add the broccoli rabe and salt, then sauté for about 3 minutes.
4. Add the water, cover, and allow to steam for about 2 minutes. Check for desired tenderness.
5. If needed, add a bit more water and allow it to steam for a few more minutes.
6. Adjust the salt and pepper if desired.

7

SNACKS

SNACKING FASCINATES ME. You're right, it's a strange thing to be interested in, but as a nutritionist and health writer, I spend a lot of time talking and writing about snacking—the pros and cons—what makes a healthful snack, what snacking does to or for your health, and such. And while I am not enthusiastically pro-snacking, detoxing can be a hungry business, so I support the desire to graze.

But—yes, there is a *but*—you have no business nibbling packaged snack foods while detoxing. I know you already know that, but I just want to make sure you understand that if you choose to eat between meals while on the 7-Day Superfood Cleanse, it must be on whole foods. No chips or crisps or crackers or cookies or (heaven forbid!) candy or cereal bars. These items aren't the most supportive choices for health or weight loss at any point, but they are absolute no-nos while detoxing.

The snackers among you may be feeling a bit nervous right now. I want to allay your fears: You can still graze. But please make sure you stick with one of the snacks in this chapter. Think of this as an adventure in eating a new way! I am very excited that you have this opportunity to see food in a different guise—not as something to alleviate boredom, but as a deeply nourishing gift to your body and soul. (Those of you who are politically minded may be interested to know that by choosing whole foods, you are *not* contributing to the $374 billion global snack industry—according to the 2014 *Nielsen Global Survey of Snacking*.)

CREAMY TREATS

I thought about calling this short section "Chia Treats" because both recipes in it contain chia, but decided that you'd be more likely to keep reading if I hooked you with the word "creamy." Because, let's face it, while some of us love to crunch, others of us love to bliss out with creamy foods. Unfortunately, most creamy foods are not cleanse-friendly! But chia, which becomes soft and gel-like when exposed to liquids, is out-rageously detox-supportive—and nutritious, thanks to protein, fiber, omega-3 fatty acids, minerals, and vitamins!

The two recipes in this section are great, non-sweet treats that have a nice, creamy mouthfeel. If you haven't had chia before, keep reading to learn more. Some of you will adore it immediately. Others of you may need to try it a few times before you get used to its tapioca-like texture.

TAP INTO THE POWER OF CHIA

Are you feeling alive, vibrant, healthy, focused? Like you can accomplish anything? As the co-author of *Chia: The Complete Guide to the Ultimate Superfood* (Sterling, 2012), I am definitely biased, but I think chia is one of the most important—and easiest—superfoods to add to your everyday diet. It makes every-thing from your hair to your skin look better. It helps prevent and treat health conditions such as diabetes, hypertension, high cholesterol, depression, and anxiety. And it lubricates muscles and joints so you can exercise more, better, and safer—and recover faster.

CHIA FRESCA

I'd like to teach you how to make Chia Fresca, an easy way to get your daily dose of that beauty-boosting, body-bettering, energy infusing superfood, chia. I know this is a drink, but the reason it's not in the drink section is that I (and my detoxers) use it as a snack. When it's mixed with liquid, chia's natural soluble fiber swells, creating a tummy-filling drink that squelches your urge to overeat. It's a great tool to use before parties and restaurant dinners to ensure you don't overeat.

Some people (usually those who like tapioca pudding and bubble tea) love its soft-jelly/slightly-crunchy texture. Others are just grossed out by it. Try a glass and see what you think.

> 1–2 tablespoons of whole chia seed (either black or white is fine, although black has a slightly higher antioxidant content, making it my first choice)
> Water to fill one large glass, about 8 ounces
> Optional: A squirt (about 1 tablespoon) of lemon or lime

1. Place the chia seeds in the bottom of a drinking glass.
2. Slowly add water, stirring as you fill the glass.
3. Allow the seeds to stand for 2–3 minutes, stirring occasionally to break up clumps. Add citrus juice, if using.
4. Stir once (or twice) before drinking.
5. Enjoy!

CHIA PUDDING
MAKES 2 SERVINGS

Protein-rich chia provides an easy, steady supply of energy that works as well for the average person, trying to get through the day, as it does for an endurance athlete. To experience the benefits of chia, may I suggest something sweet and delicious—like this chia pudding recipe made with coconut? It makes a lovely afternoon snack. It's also a great way to start the day: My kids sometimes have this for breakfast with a green drink.

⅔ cup chia seeds
2 cups canned or fresh coconut milk
½ teaspoon vanilla extract
Optional sweetener: Just a drizzle of coconut nectar, honey, maple syrup, or other natural sweetener
Optional topping: 2 tablespoons unsweetened coconut flakes or 1 tablespoon chopped nuts or seeds

1. Put chia seeds, coconut milk, vanilla, and, if using, optional sweetener, in a 1-quart glass jar with a lid. Tighten the lid and shake well to combine thoroughly, or stir the ingredients in a bowl to combine.

2. Allow the pudding to thicken for 30 minutes or more. (Or, even better, make the pudding in the evening and let it sit, covered, overnight in the fridge.)

3. Adjust liquid if necessary. Spoon the pudding into bowls and top with optional coconut or nuts, if desired.

SNACKING: DID YOU KNOW. . .?

- Forty-eight percent of consumers in the United States snack at least twice a day, up from 25 percent in 2010.*
- Ninety-one percent of consumers polled say they snack at least once a day. And 21 percent are snacking three or four times daily—the majority of whom are women.**
- Sales of packaged snack food in the United States are expected to reach $22.9 billion in 2016 .*
- A 2010 study showed that children in the United States snacked, on average, six times per day, approximately twice as often as American children in the 1970s.*
- Sixty-three percent of Americans surveyed said they'd snacked on some sort of chip within the past 30 days. Sixty-four percent of those surveyed in fifty-nine countries outside North America said they'd snacked on fruit in the past thirty days.**
- Annual snack food sales across the world are Europe ($167 billion), North America ($124 billion), Asia-Pacific ($46 billion), Latin America ($30 billion) and the Middle East/Africa ($7 billion).**
- Confections—which include sugary sweets like chocolate, hard candy, and gum—comprise the biggest sales contribution to the overall snack category in Europe ($46.5 billion) and the Middle East/Africa ($1.9 billion).**
- Salty snacks make up more than one-fifth of snack sales in North America ($27.7 billion).**
- Refrigerated snacks comprise almost one third of snacks in Asia-Pacific ($13.7 billion).**
- Cookies and snack cakes make up more than one fourth of total snacks in Latin America ($8.6 billion).**

*Source: Technomic's *Snacking Occasion Consumer Trend Report* for 2014.
**Source: *2014 Nielsen Global Survey of Snacking.*

VEGGIES

Ah, veggies, my favorite food category on the planet, and probably the most undereaten. This is a shame because not only do vegetables taste amazing, they are filled with important phytonutrients, vitamins, minerals, fiber, protein, and other good things, most which are very alkalizing—making them great for detoxers. Vegetables fill you up and make you look and feel amazing. They are a boon to detoxers, because they help squash the powerful carb and caffeine cravings so many of us have (the ones that are often so strong that we just can't resist them). Without these cravings, staying on a healthy food plan is so much easier!

CRUDITÉS

MAKES 1–2 SERVINGS

When I was an older teen, I used to come to New York City each summer to work. I was a small-town farm girl, staying with my big city, opera-singing aunt. Everything she did, said, and served felt exotic to me. It was in her Central Park West apartment that I first heard the word *crudités*—to describe a platter of endive spears, raw strips of bell pepper, jicama slices, broccoli and cauliflower florets, halved radishes, carrot and celery sticks, and slices of fennel. Growing up, I ate very few raw vegetables: Once in a while my parents would put out a sliced beefsteak tomato or some freshly pulled spring onions with a plate of salt.

So why am I telling you this story? Because crudités are the ultimate detox food: The raw veggies are alkalizing, full of helpful fiber, nutrient-dense, and detoxifying. If you can, enjoy them with almond or cashew butter or a protein-rich hummus or bean-based dip.

If this sounds boring to you, then I challenge you to go out and find some new veggies to crunch on. Go ahead and use one of the superfood detoxifying dips in this chapter. Enjoy!

1. Wash your veggies of choice and pat dry.
2. Peel, slice, or cut your chosen vegetables in any way that you fancy.

CRUNCHY THINGS

We love to crunch, don't we? You can admit it! I can't judge any of you because I am a cruncher as well (tortilla chips are my weakness). Crunching is a proprioceptive activity. Proprioceptive means "stimuli that is created and perceived within the body, especially those connected with the position and movement of the body." In other words, crunching provides a lot of what occupational therapists call "input" to your jaw. People find this both calming and stimulating, making it a very satisfying activity!

The bad thing about crunching, however, is that so many of the things we choose to chomp on aren't great for our health. I'm talking about chips, crackers, pretzels, Cheez Doodles, and the like. Fortunately, Mother Nature has created some delicious munchies that will not only give our jaws the workout they want, but will supply us with the nutrients we need to get (and stay) healthy, while supplying a natural detox for our bodies.

SNACKING DEFINED

Snack: A small amount of food eaten between meals. The word first appeared in the English language around 1759 and is thought to come from the Middle English word *snak*, to bite. As a verb, the word *snack* means to eat a small amount of food between meals.

COCONUT CHIPS
USING A MATURE COCONUT
MAKES 4 SERVINGS

This recipe comes from my latest cookbook, *Coconut: The Complete Guide to the World's Most Versatile Superfood* (Sterling, 2015). You can buy a small bag of coconut chips at the supermarket, or you can make your own.

Dogs love these chips, so guard them well if you happen to be a pet owner who doesn't want to share.

1 mature coconut
Coarse salt

1. Preheat oven to 350°F.
2. Test each of the three eyes at the stem end of coconut to see which two are the softest. Then use a clean ice pick, screwdriver, or large nail and a clean hammer to pierce these two soft eyes. (You can also pierce soft eyes with a corkscrew.)
3. Strain the coconut water through a fine sieve into a bowl; reserve it for other uses (there are plenty of ideas in this book—just look under *coconut* in the index).
4. Place the whole coconut on a rimmed baking sheet and bake for 30 minutes, or until the coconut shell begins to crack. Set the coconut aside until it is cool enough to handle.
5. Wrap the coconut in a clean kitchen towel, place it on a stable surface, and hit it with a hammer in the same place several times to crack the outer shell and split the coconut into several large pieces.
6. Separate the coconut flesh from shell and use a vegetable peeler to remove the dark outer skin, if desired.
7. Using a sharp paring knife or a vegetable peeler, shave coconut meat into strips.
8. Rinse the coconut strips in a colander, then spread them in a single layer on a kitchen towel to dry.
9. Divide the coconut strips between two rimmed baking sheets in a single layer. Season with salt.
10. Bake until toasted, about 10 minutes.

ROASTED COCONUT CHICKPEAS

MAKES 4 SERVINGS

Roasted chickpeas are an easy-to-make, protein-rich, fiber-filled, outrageously healthy snack. This recipe is flexible: increase the salt by a couple pinches, and add your favorite savory spices, such as cumin or rosemary.

1 15-ounce can chickpeas, rinsed and drained (or 2 cups cooked)
1 tablespoon liquid coconut oil
½ teaspoon salt
1 teaspoon ground cinnamon or ½ teaspoon allspice
Pinch of black pepper (optional)

1. Preheat oven to 450°F.
2. Thoroughly dry the chickpeas with paper towels. If necessary, aim a blow dryer, set to low or cool, on the chickpeas to help get rid of any excess moisture. The beans need to be dry.
3. Place dry chickpeas in a single layer on one or two baking trays. Roast for 15 minutes.
4. Remove from the oven and, while still warm, toss in a large bowl with the coconut oil, salt, spice, and, if desired, pepper, making sure all chickpeas are fully coated.
5. Return the chickpeas to the baking trays and place in the oven. Roast for an additional 15–20 minutes until crunchy and golden.

BAKED KALE CHIPS

SERVES 4

These kale chips are a delicious, low-calorie, nutritious snack, and, like potato chips, you cannot stop at eating just one. *Baked Kale Chips* are loaded with vitamins, minerals, phytonutrients, and fiber. They're great for parties and starting a conversation. Try them! This recipe comes from my book, *Kale: A Complete Guide to the World's Most Powerful Superfood* (Sterling, 2013).

1 bunch kale
2 teaspoons extra-virgin olive oil or coconut oil
1 teaspoon seasoned salt

1. Preheat the oven to 350°F.
2. Line a non-insulated cookie sheet with parchment paper.
3. With a knife or kitchen shears carefully remove the leaves from the thick stems (save the stems to use in your juicer!) and tear them into bite-size pieces. Wash and thoroughly dry the kale in a salad spinner. Drizzle the kale with olive oil and sprinkle with seasoned salt.
4. Bake for 5 minutes, then turn the kale leaves.
5. Bake the leaves another 5–10 minutes, until the edges are brown but not burned. Allow the kale chips to cool on a baking sheet before serving.

SALT AND VINEGAR KALE CHIPS
SERVES 4

In this snack recipe, crispy baked kale is seasoned with vinegar and salt—a great, healthy stand-in for commercial salt and vinegar chips.

1 bunch kale
2 teaspoons extra-virgin olive oil or coconut oil, divided
1 teaspoon sherry vinegar
1 pinch sea salt, to taste

1. Preheat the oven to 300°F.
2. Cut away the inner ribs from each kale leaf and discard or save to use in your juicer. Tear the leaves into pieces of uniform size. (I make my pieces about the size of a small potato chip.) Wash the torn kale pieces and spin dry in a salad spinner or dry with paper towels until they're very dry.
3. Put the kale pieces in a large resealable bag (or use a bowl if you don't mind getting your hands oily). Add about half of the olive oil, then seal and squeeze the bag to evenly distribute the oil among the kale pieces. Add the remaining oil and squeeze the bag a bit more, until all kale pieces are evenly coated with oil and lightly massaged.
4. Sprinkle the vinegar over the kale leaves, reseal the bag, and then shake it to distribute the vinegar evenly over the leaves. Spread the leaves onto a baking sheet in a single layer.
5. Bake for 5 minutes, then turn the kale leaves.
6. Roast the leaves for another 15–20 minutes, or until mostly crisp. Season with salt and serve immediately.

WHAT STEPHANIE LIKES TO SNACK ON

This may seem like a funny thing to say in a chapter on snack recipes, but you don't need specially designated "snack foods" in order to enjoy healthy food between meals. In fact, I rarely eat snack foods. When I'm hungry and can't wait until the next meal, I just head for the fridge for a small portion of whatever leftovers are there, or I grab a handful of nuts or seeds (sunflower and pumpkin are my favorite) or warm up a cup of soup. Here are some of my favorite non-snack, detox-friendly snack foods:

- A glass of tomato juice or vegetable cocktail. Sometimes I'll warm it up with a bit of minced garlic for a quick soup.
- A small green drink, pink drink, or watermelon cooler (see the recipes in chapter 4)
- A cup of veggie broth
- A cup of vegan chili
- A cup of puréed vegetable soup
- A cup of vegan curry (all-vegetable, no grain)
- A small portion of anything I ate last night. I use a tea saucer–size plate to keep my portion small.
- A baked artichoke (leaves and heart)
- A cup of roasted or sautéed veggies
- 1 cup of salsa, eaten with a fork if thick, or a spoon if thin
- A small salad
- A cup of beans, either as-is or dressed with a chopped scallion and a tablespoon of salsa or pesto
- A carrot, grated and dressed with a half tablespoon of dressing. Sometimes I throw on a few chopped nuts or seeds.

DIPS

I am a mother. I mention this because I often learn things "on the job" as I parent and feed my three sons that benefit my clients. What I have been taught again and again by my kids is that if I want my clients to eat veggies, I need to give them something fun to eat *with* the veggies. Enter dip. I love dips that contain brain-and-heart-supportive fats, vitamins, minerals, fiber, protein, amino acids, and phytonutrients—all of which help you lose weight, strengthen your health, fight cravings, boost your looks, and support your immune system while tasting great! Every single dip in this chapter is beneficial for detoxing. Enjoy!

RAW ZUCCHINI HUMMUS
MAKES A LITTLE MORE THAN 1 CUP

This fun raw food version of hummus contains no chickpeas. It's a great way to use up zucchini (you gardeners will know how important this is!) or another type of summer squash.

> 1 cup peeled and chopped zucchini or other variety of summer squash
> ¼ cup lemon juice
> 2 tablespoons olive oil
> 2 big cloves of garlic
> 1 teaspoons salt
> A pinch of smoked paprika
> ½ cup raw tahini* (or regular tahini), stirred well before measured

1. Add all ingredients except for the tahini to a food processor. Blend until smooth.
2. Add the tahini and blend until smooth.

*Raw tahini is made with raw sesame seeds. Regular tahini is typically made with sesame seeds that have been toasted.

HUMMUS
MAKES ABOUT 2½ CUPS

Hummus is so easy to make that I encourage you to make your own (it tastes even fresher and better than the commercial stuff). If you don't have time to make your own, however, or prefer store-bought hummus, do your body a favor and check the ingredient list before you toss it into your shopping cart. Go for a brand that uses all olive oil and no soybean oil (this cheap oil is not good for detoxing), and is made without additives (such as potassium sorbate, a preservative that extends products' shelf life and may damage DNA, according to some sources). If you want to make your own hummus, but don't like tahini, you can leave it out—the hummus will be a little runnier, but it's not a big deal; it'll still taste delicious. Oh, and feel free to flavor this hummus recipe with chipotle paste, puréed roasted red peppers, herbs, pesto, olive tapenade... or whatever seasoning you like.

> 2 cups drained, well cooked or canned chickpeas, liquid reserved
> ½ cup tahini (stir well before measuring)
> ¼ cup extra-virgin olive oil, plus oil for drizzling
> 2 cloves garlic, peeled (use more if you'd like; garlic is detoxifying!)
> Salt and freshly ground black pepper, to taste
> 1 or more teaspoons ground cumin
> Juice of 1 lemon, plus more as needed

1. Put all the ingredients except the reserved chickpea liquid in a food processor and process. Pulse in a small amount of the chickpea liquid or water at a time, as needed, to help create a smooth purée.
2. Taste and adjust the seasoning.
3. Store in a covered container in the refrigerator.

WHITE BEAN DIP
MAKES ABOUT 1¼ CUPS

White bean dip is made the same way hummus is, but it has a milder, creamier flavor. When I am not detoxing, I even use it as a substitute for mayonnaise or dairy products. Play with this one. Toss in a bit of caramelized onion or roasted garlic if you like. Change up the herbs and spices. Purée your favorite veggie and stir it in. You get the idea!

2 cups cooked or canned cannellini (white kidney beans), drained
1½ tablespoons fresh lemon juice
1½ tablespoons extra-virgin olive oil
1 large garlic clove, peeled
¾ teaspoon ground cumin
Salt and pepper, to taste
1 tablespoon of chopped dill, chives, parsley, or other herbs
   (optional)

1. Puree the first five ingredients in a food processor. Process until almost smooth.
2. Season with salt and pepper. Transfer the dip to a small bowl.
3. Stir in optional chopped herbs by hand.

AVOCADO-COCONUT DIP
MAKES ABOUT 1½ CUPS

I think of this dip as "coconut-kissed" guacamole. It is filled with healthy fats from both the avocado and the coconut cream, making it a nourishing (and delicious) superfood dip.

> 3 tablespoons coconut cream or coconut milk, at room
>   temperature
> 1 tablespoon fresh lemon or lime juice
> 1 ripe avocado
> Salt, to taste
> Black pepper, to taste

1. In a small bowl, thoroughly mix the coconut cream and lemon juice.
2. In a separate bowl, mash the avocado until smooth.
3. Mix the avocado into the coconut-lemon mixture and season to taste with salt and pepper.

EASY PUMPKIN PROTEIN DIP
MAKES 1½ CUPS

You can dress up purchased or homemade hummus with pumpkin and a bit of spice! Take my word for it, this recipe, based on one in my book *The Pumpkin Pie Spice Cookbook* (Sterling, 2014), is delicious and particularly lovely with veggies.

> 1 8-ounce container hummus (or 1 cup of homemade hummus)
> ¼ cup pumpkin purée
> ¼ teaspoon pumpkin pie spice

1. Stir together all ingredients until well blended.

GARLICKY KALE AND SPINACH DIP

MAKES ABOUT 2 CUPS

This glorious superfood dip is vegan, low-cal, and filled with antioxidants and powerful phytonutrients. Make this often—it's as delicious as it is virtuous.

> 1 cup cooked or steamed chopped kale, squeezed dry
> 1 cup cooked or steamed spinach, squeezed dry
> 2 medium garlic cloves, peeled
> 3 tablespoons toasted pine nuts (or use almonds if you'd like)
> 4 teaspoons balsamic vinegar
> ⅓ cup olive oil
> Salt and pepper to taste

1. Add the kale and spinach to the bowl of a food processor. Pulse until puréed.
2. Add the garlic, pine nuts, and vinegar. Pulse to purée, slowly adding in the olive oil.
3. Scrape down the bowl, add salt and pepper, and pulse to blend.

8

DINNER

IN THE WORLD OF CLEANSES, DINNER is a small affair. Depending upon the particular detox program, it can be a glass of water with lemon, a cup of tea, a green drink, a cup of soup, or a salad. In other words, it's considerably smaller than what most of us eat in our everyday lives.

There's a reason for this. Your body's systems begin to slow down toward the end of the day, which results in a lower body temperature and drowsiness. Eating larger amounts of food later in the day, when your body is readying for sleep, can lead to inefficient digestion. It also makes it difficult for the body to detoxify.

Hence the small detox dinners you will find in this chapter. Take a look and you'll find a lot of salads and a lot of soup (soy-free, dairy-free, wheat-free, and meat-free), plus some of my favorite salad dressings.

Enjoy soup or salad. If you're really hungry, you can have both, but don't have more than that—and refrain from adding animal ingredients, sugars, or lots of protein—because it will derail your detox. The light soup and salad recipes in this chapter have been developed to keep you deeply nourished and move through your system quickly, in

ARE ALL CALORIES EQUAL?

While some medical experts believe a calorie is a calorie is a calorie, regardless of when you eat it, holistic practitioners tend to believe that the later you eat, the lighter you should eat. This was recently borne out by a study performed by researchers at Northwestern University, who found that eating later at night led to twice as much weight gain—even when total calories consumed were the same.

order to help flush out water weight and toxins while you sleep. The result? You'll look and feel better—and thinner. If you find you are still hungry, have a second helping of soup or salad, or pull out your blender or juicer and enjoy a green drink nightcap!

SOUPS

I am the grandchild of farmers who ate large breakfasts and midday meals, and who then came in from the fields at the end of the day to a bowl of soup and maybe a piece of bread and a piece of fruit. This is the same meal that many people in cultures all over the world enjoy each night. There is much wisdom in making dinner a light, liquid meal: Most of us don't do a lot of moving around in the evening, so we really do not need a lot of calories. In addition, toward the end of the day, our body systems begin to slow down in service to a night of deep, refreshing sleep. When there's a lot of dense food sitting in your stomach waiting to be digested, sleep can be disrupted. If you're on the 7-Day Superfood Cleanse, you'll want to keep your evening meal light and liquid for an additional reason: When you make it easy for your body to digest the evening meal before sleep, your body can concentrate on flushing out trapped water weight and toxins while you are in dreamland.

The soups in this chapter are some of my clients' favorites (mine, too). You'll also find the *Dinner Soup Blueprint*, which will give you choices for making a variety of fun, nourishing, superfood-filled soups based on what you have in the house. Have fun with it! If you're not a cook, go ahead and pick up high-quality, premade vegan soups that do not contain meat. I know dinner will feel like a small meal for most of you, but give it a try. If you are still hungry, go ahead and have another bowl of soup or make a small salad to enjoy—or treat yourself to a green smoothie (page 54) or green drink (page 56).

DINNER SOUP BLUEPRINT
MAKES ABOUT 4 SERVINGS

Cooking is definitely my thing. I have always loved playing in the kitchen. I've been to culinary school and worked as a kitchen assistant and cooking teacher. These days, I'm a practicing nutritionist and write cookbooks. I rarely follow recipes anymore; instead I enjoy creating something delicious from ingredients I have on hand. Not everyone feels comfortable with cooking that way, however, which is why I've developed the *Dinner Soup Blueprint*. It's a loose recipe that allows you to make a detox-friendly, superfood-filled dinner soup that will not only nourish you but also encourage your body to release trapped water, toxins, and weight. Play with it, using your favorite vegetables, herbs, and beans. It is the ultimate dinner food. Enjoy yourself!

1 tablespoon extra-virgin olive oil or coconut oil
1 stalk celery, chopped
1 large onion, chopped
2–4 large garlic cloves, minced
2 cups chopped green, orange, or red vegetables, chopped
6 cups vegetable broth
1 can (about 2 cups cooked) white beans, rinsed and drained
Salt and pepper to taste
A dash of curry powder, chili powder, cumin, or any other spices,
   or 1–3 teaspoons chopped fresh herb of choice (optional)

1. Heat the oil in a large pot over medium heat. Add the celery, onion, and garlic. Stir until softened, about 5 minutes.
2. Add your chosen vegetables to the pot and stir until softened, about 5 minutes.
3. Add the vegetable broth, beans, salt and pepper, and chosen spices or herbs. Allow to cook for a minute or two longer, to blend.
4. Working in batches, pour the soup into a blender until the blender pitcher is no more than half full. Purée the soup until completely smooth, and return the puréed soup to the pot. Continue until all the soup is blended. Alternatively, use a stick blender to purée the soup in the pot.

SPICY PUMPKIN COCONUT BISQUE

MAKES ABOUT 4 SERVINGS

Light, deeply nutritious, delicious, and just exotic enough to be exciting, this pumpkin soup is fantastic and easy. It freezes well, too—if you have any leftovers. This is adapted from my book *The Pumpkin Pie Spice Cookbook* (Sterling, 2014).

> 1 tablespoon extra-virgin olive oil or coconut oil
> 1 large onion, chopped
> 1 or 2 large garlic cloves, minced
> 2 cups vegetable broth
> 2 14-ounce cans pumpkin purée
> 1 14-ounce can regular coconut milk
> 2 tablespoons orange or lemon juice
> 2 teaspoons ground ginger
> 2 teaspoons pumpkin pie spice
> 2 teaspoons chili powder

1. Heat the oil in a large pot over medium heat. Add the onion and garlic. Stir until softened, about 5 minutes.

2. Add the broth to the onion and garlic. Cook 2–3 minutes.

3. Stir the pumpkin purée, coconut milk, orange juice, ginger, pumpkin pie spice, and chili powder into the liquid. Bring the soup to a simmer and cook until heated through, 5 to 7 minutes.

4. Working in batches, pour the soup into a blender until the blender pitcher is no more than half full. Purée the soup until completely smooth, and return the puréed soup to the pot. Continue until all the soup is blended. Alternatively, use a stick blender to purée the soup in the pot.

5. Warm the puréed soup over medium heat. Bring to a simmer and cook another 10 minutes.

SUPERFOOD BEET SOUP
MAKES 4 SERVINGS

Beets are a common detox ingredient, because they contain betaine, a nutrient that helps your body excrete toxins. And yet, I am always surprised by people who simply don't eat beets, even if they haven't prepared them themselves or, through lack or exposure, aren't entirely sure if they like or dislike them. If this is you (and even if it is not you!) please try this recipe. Not only is it delicious, it is fun! If you like, leave out the ginger and add a hot pepper, cumin or cilantro, or lime juice—or all three—to create a more Mexican flavor profile.

1 tablespoon coconut oil or extra virgin olive oil
1 large onion, diced
3 cloves garlic, finely chopped
1 tablespoon finely chopped ginger
3 large red beets, peeled and cut into ¼-inch pieces
5 cups vegetable stock, divided
1 14-ounce can coconut milk
½ teaspoon salt
¼ teaspoon freshly ground black pepper
Chopped chives, dill, or parsley, for garnish (optional)

1. In a large pot, heat the oil over medium heat. Sauté the onion for 5 minutes.
2. Add the garlic and ginger. Cook, stirring often, for 5 minutes.
3. Add the beets and 4 cups of the stock. Bring to a boil, then reduce the heat and simmer until the beets are fork-tender, about 20 minutes.
4. With an immersion blender, or working in batches with a regular blender, purée the soup, adding the remaining 1 cup of stock, as needed, to reach the desired consistency.
5. Stir in the coconut milk, salt, and pepper.
6. Garnish with herbs, if desired.

CARROT SOUP
MAKES ABOUT 6½ CUPS

This refreshing soup can be eaten chilled, at room temperature, or warm. I prefer it warm, but it is so delicious and healthy (it contains tons of beta-carotene for great skin and eyesight) that I'll take it however I can get it.

2 tablespoons coconut oil or extra virgin olive oil
1 shallot, finely chopped
1 small onion, chopped
1 tablespoon finely grated peeled fresh ginger root
1 tablespoon mild curry powder
4 cups chopped carrots
2½ cups broth
Salt and pepper, to taste
1–1½ cups canned coconut milk
1 tablespoon fresh lime juice, plus additional to taste
Water for thinning soup
Chopped scallions or herb of choice, for garnish (optional)

1. In a large heavy saucepan, heat the coconut oil over medium heat. Add the shallot, onion, ginger root, and curry powder and cook until the shallot and onion are tender.
2. Add the carrots, broth, and salt and pepper, and simmer until the carrots are very tender, about 20 minutes.
3. With an immersion blender, or working in batches with a regular blender, purée the soup with the coconut milk and lime juice until very smooth.
4. Adjust salt and pepper, if needed, and thin with water if necessary.
5. If serving the soup warm, allow it to cool to just above room temperature and ladle into soup bowls. Serve garnished with chopped scallions or herbs, if desired.
6. If serving the soup cold, transfer it to an airtight container and place it in the refrigerator. This soup actually tastes best the second day, so I usually make it the day before and stash it in the fridge so I can garnish and serve it the next day.

SIMPLE TOMATO SOUP
MAKES 6 SERVINGS

For me, tomato soup is comfort food. My mother couldn't cook, so most of the food we ate growing up came out of boxes, bags, and cans. Campbell's cream of tomato soup was one of our favorites. Now that my palate is a bit more sophisticated (emphasis on *a bit*), I prefer my tomato soup homemade. If you don't like a lot of spice, you can remove some or all of it from this recipe, and you'll still get a beautiful bowl of soup.

4 tablespoons coconut oil or extra virgin olive
2 medium yellow onions, chopped
1 teaspoon salt
3 teaspoons curry powder
1 teaspoon ground coriander
1 teaspoon ground cumin
½ teaspoon red chile pepper flakes
2 28-ounce cans whole tomatoes, juice reserved
4 cups chicken or vegetable broth
1 14-ounce can coconut milk
Black pepper, to taste (optional)

1. Add coconut oil to a large pot over medium heat. Add the onions and salt, and cook, stirring occasionally, until the onions are very soft, about 10 minutes.
2. Stir in the curry powder, coriander, cumin, and chile flakes, and cook, stirring constantly, about 30 seconds, or until spices are fragrant.
3. Stir in the tomatoes, the juice from the cans, and 4 cups of broth. Simmer for 15 minutes or until the flavors have blended.
4. With an immersion blender, or working in batches with a regular blender, purée the soup with the coconut milk until very smooth.
5. Adjust the seasonings and, if desired, add black pepper.

DINNER SALADS

During the 7-Day Superfood Cleanse, your dinner will be soup, salad, or both. Yes, you read that correctly. For a week, you'll "go light at night," as I like to say to my clients. The salads in this section are some of my favorites. All of them make fantastic dinners, either eaten alone or paired with a soup and/or a green drink. Feel free to mix them up a bit and add in your favorite veggies or use more of one ingredient or another. The *Dinner Salad Blueprint* allows you to create an easy, customized salad every single night of the detox, should you choose to experiment. For those of you who don't like making your own food or don't have the time, order from a restaurant or go to a salad bar. Just skip dairy, animal-based, wheat-based, sweet, fruity, or otherwise non-cleanse-friendly ingredients.

EVENING COCKTAILS
AND OTHER ALCOHOLIC BEVERAGES

I know how important the after-work cocktail, beer, or glass of wine is for many of you—me, too! But alcohol greatly inhibits your body's ability to detoxify, shed water bloat, lose weight, and maintain weight loss when you drink nightly. I love my glass of wine as much as the next woman, but for the duration of the 7-Day Superfood Cleanse, you'll need to let go of alcohol.

Once you're off the cleanse, your best bet is to limit yourself to four alcoholic drinks a week—not daily. For those of you who drink, watching your alcohol intake will set you up for the biggest success with weight loss and renewed good health.

If you feel that you need something festive to drink in the evening, break out the other bubbly (seltzer), put it in a sexy glass, dress it up with lemon or lime, and make a toast to your health! Skoal!

DINNER SALAD BLUEPRINT
MAKES 2 SERVINGS

Salads don't need to be fussy to be fantastic. This is a recipe that can be played with in an infinite number of ways, so feel free to experiment and create something different at each meal!

3 tablespoons coconut vinegar or apple cider vinegar
3 tablespoons coconut aminos (or use wheat-free natural soy sauce)
1½ tablespoons extra virgin olive oil, or liquid coconut oil
1 teaspoon coconut sugar (optional)
1 teaspoon mustard of choice (optional)
Salt and pepper, to taste
8–9 cups salad greens of choice
1 cup chopped vegetable(s) of choice
2 cups cooked beans or lentils or dried peas (or use ⅓ cup of chopped nuts or seeds)
¼ cup chopped fresh herbs (optional)

1. In a large bowl, whisk together the vinegar, coconut aminos, oil, coconut sugar (if desired), mustard (if desired), and salt and pepper.
2. Add the salad greens, chopped vegetables, beans, and herbs, if you like, to the bowl. Toss until all ingredients are coated with dressing. Serve immediately.

CHOPPED AVOCADO COCONUT SALAD
MAKES 2 SERVINGS

There are people in my life who don't like salad. Can you believe it? They complain that salads are too leafy and, certainly, too green, too fiber-filled, or just plain boring. They go on to say that the dressing is too acidic or too this or too that. But not a single salad hater I know can resist a good chopped salad. This one happens to be one of my absolute favorites. It's filled with superfoods, and it's just exotic enough to hold people's interest. Try it! I bet you'll love it as much as I do!

1 large Hass avocado, halved and pitted
1½ tablespoons fresh lime juice
1½ teaspoons Asian chili-garlic sauce, such as Sriracha
3 tablespoons liquid coconut oil or extra virgin olive oil
Salt and pepper, to taste
2 cups cooked beans or lentils (or use ⅓ cup chopped nuts)
1 cup diced peeled jicama
1 cup diced red onion
1 large red bell pepper, diced
¼ cup unsweetened shredded dried coconut
¼ cup chopped cashews
¼ cup chopped fresh cilantro
7 cups chopped romaine lettuce
Salad dressing of choice

1. Scoop the avocado flesh into a food processor or blender. Add the lime juice, chili-garlic sauce, and coconut oil, and process until smooth. Season generously with salt and pepper.
2. In a large bowl, toss together the remaining ingredients.
3. If you are eating right away, pour the dressing over the salad and toss, toss, toss, until all ingredients are coated in dressing. If you are taking the salad to work, pack the dressing separately and dress the salad right before eating.

CELERIAC AND BEET SALAD

This salad recipe is little different than the usual because it uses root veggies as a base, which I absolutely love. Feel free to substitute kohlrabi for the beet or carrot, if you like, or swap in jicama for the celeriac. Try this recipe once, as written, and then get ready to experiment!

1 large carrot, peeled
1 medium beet, peeled
½ large celeriac (also known as celery root), ends trimmed and
   peeled
2 tablespoons fresh mint leaves, minced (substitute cilantro if
   you'd like)
Juice of 1 medium lemon or lime
1 tablespoon extra-virgin olive oil
Salt and pepper to taste
½ cup sunflower seeds

1. Using a box grater or a grater attachment on your food processor, finely shred the carrot, beet, and celeriac. Stir in the mint leaves. Set aside.

2. In a large bowl, whisk together the lemon juice, olive oil, salt, and pepper.

3. Dump in the shredded vegetables and toss to coat.

4. Adjust the salt and pepper and top with sunflower seeds.

NUTTY KALE SALAD

MAKES 6 SERVINGS

I first tasted kale salad at my brother and sister-in-law's house and fell in love with it instantly! Not only does this salad taste great, it makes me feel wonderful and strong after eating it. It is also one of those recipes that people will ask for, so feel free to share it. The recipe is adapted from my book *Kale: The Complete Guide to the World's Most Powerful Superfood* (Sterling, 2013). Feel free to substitute regular green cabbage or Napa cabbage for the kale.

> 1 cup chopped almonds or sunflower seeds, divided
> 2 tablespoons cilantro leaves (optional)
> ⅓ cup extra virgin olive oil or liquid coconut oil
> ⅓ cup apple cider vinegar (or you can use lemon juice)
> 1 tablespoon agave syrup or honey
> Salt and pepper to taste
> A few shakes of Tabasco or other hot sauce (optional)
> 2 large bunches kale, about 2 pounds, de-ribbed and cut in a chiffonade*
> 2 orange or red bell peppers, cleaned and cut into very fine strips
> 1 large carrot, peeled and shredded (use a box grater or a food processor with a grater attachment)

1. In a food processor, pulse together ¼ cup of the nuts, cilantro, oil, vinegar, agave, salt, pepper and hot sauce. Pulse until nuts are half pureed. Set aside.

2. In a large bowl, toss together the kale, bell pepper, carrots, and the remaining nuts or seeds.

3. Using a spatula to get every last drop, scrape the dressing over the kale mixture. Toss to coat the vegetables evenly.

4. Allow the salad to sit for 20 minutes to blend the flavors before serving.

Chiffonade means *little ribbons* in French. This cutting technique creates long, thin, beautiful strips from leafy veggies. To create this effect, make a stack of leaves (cabbage, collards, chard, spinach, a salad green, basil leaves, or any other culinary green). Roll the stack tightly into a cigar shape, then slice the roll on an angle.

COMING DOWN FROM THE DAY

For many detoxers, daytime is easy: They put themselves on auto-pilot and follow cleanse instructions while also getting everything else done—all without a lot of thought. However, once the sun goes down, things get dicey.

Evening is a time for relaxing, vegging out, and having all the fun you didn't get to experience during your workday. But it is also a time to preserve your energy and, at the same time, create more energy for the next day—all while supporting nighttime needs for reflection and rest.

I have found in my life, and in the lives of my clients, that when it comes to energy, you can do everything right during the day but make choices in the evening that completely cancel out your daytime commitment to creating and sustaining healthy energy levels.

If you want detoxing to work for you—and gain all the benefits you set out to gain—now is the time to focus and commit to making more energy-supportive evening choices. These after-dinner activities will feed your soul so you'll be less likely to distract yourself with food:

- Write in your journal or start a new one
- Make a bucket list (wish list)
- Read inspirational books
- Write poetry
- Draw/sketch
- Make a vision board
- Create a spa night at home
- Research places to go for your next holiday or vacation
- Use the time to reach out to friends and family you haven't contacted in a while because you've been too busy

SALAD DRESSINGS

For me, a salad dressing can make or break a salad. Truly. There have been times when my body was screaming out for raw leafy greens, but the only way I could get myself to eat even one leaf of arugula was to bribe myself with an amazing salad dressing. That's why I've included so many dressings here—including the fun, customizable *Creamy Salad Dressing Blueprint*. All of them are detox-friendly and feature protein, fiber, and a range of vitamins, minerals, brain- and heart-healthy fats, and more. Make a big batch of one or two of the dressings before your detox begins, or mix one up fresh as needed. They are all easy to make, deeply nourishing, and very yummy! Oh, and they're versatile, too! I've used these recipes as veggie dips and to dress up bean and grain salads.

CREAMY SALAD DRESSING BLUEPRINT

MAKE AS MUCH AS YOU WANT AND DON'T FORGET TO PLAY,
PLAY, PLAY TO MAKE THIS YOUR OWN!

By now, I guess you can tell how much I just love blueprints—probably because they appeal to my rebellious side! I like that they invite you to customize a dish based on the ingredients you have on hand, the tastes you enjoy, and the foods that make you feel the healthiest, rather than requiring you to follow a strict formula that might not appeal to your taste or fit your needs. This salad dressing blueprint is for those of you who love creamy-style salad dressings that can make even a plain lettuce salad feel substantial, but don't love all the dairy and other ingredients they contain. The nut butter in this blueprint makes it into a high-protein, high-fiber treat that you can even enjoy as a dip—try it with baby carrots.

> 1–2 tablespoons almond butter, cashew butter, sesame seed butter, or tahini
> 1 tablespoon lemon juice or vinegar of choice
> 1 tablespoon extra-virgin olive oil, avocado oil, coconut oil, rice bran oil, sesame oil, walnut oil, etc.
> 1 tablespoon hot water
> Salt, pepper, other spices
> Hot sauce (optional)
> Minced herbs, garlic, or shallots to taste

1. With a fork, mix the first three ingredients into a paste. Season with salt, pepper, hot sauce, herbs, and/or spices to taste.
2. Add hot water as needed to make the dressing the right consistency. You may need more or less hot water depending upon the consistency of the nut butter you use.

TAHINI LEMON DRESSING

MAKES ⅓ CUP

This is a great, protein-rich, creamy, savory dressing that is great for those of you who don't like vinaigrettes.

½ tablespoons tahini
¼ cup water
2 garlic cloves
3 tablespoons lemon juice
2 tablespoons tamari soy sauce
1 teaspoon maple syrup (optional)
Pinch of cayenne

1. In a blender, mix the tahini and water until combined.
2. Add the remaining ingredients and continue to mix until all ingredients are combined.
3. Adjust flavors to your taste.

MAPLE DIJON VINAIGRETTE

MAKES ABOUT ½ CUP

A classic vinaigrette, this savory/sweet dressing is perfect for a wide range of salads. Play with the vinegars and oils: This recipe is endlessly adaptable!

¼ cup apple cider, red wine, or balsamic vinegar
¼ cup extra-virgin olive oil, liquid coconut oil, or a nut oil (such as almond or hazelnut)
1 tablespoon pure maple syrup
1 tablespoon Dijon mustard
A couple pinches of sea salt and pepper

1. In a small bowl, whisk together all ingredients, or place all ingredients into a jar, cover, and shake well.
2. Cover and refrigerate.
3. Shake well before serving.

GINGER–SUNFLOWER SEED DRESSING

MAKES ABOUT 1½ CUPS

Here's another substantial, creamy, protein-rich dressing, thanks to the sunflower seeds. It's a large-batch recipe, so store any unused dressing in a tightly covered container in the fridge.

½ cup raw or roasted sunflower seeds (preferably unsalted, but salted is fine, too)
Juice of one lemon
2 tablespoons brown rice vinegar
1 tablespoon ginger root, grated
1 clove garlic
¼ cup wheat-free soy sauce
1 tablespoon honey, agave nectar, or pure maple syrup
1 cup sesame oil (feel free to cut this with extra-virgin olive oil)
2 teaspoons mustard

1. Put all ingredients into a blender and purée until smooth.
2. Refrigerate before using.

9

DETOX SELF-CARE

A cleanse is a time of cleaning out your body and cleaning up your diet so you can look and feel your best. In short, it's a time of exquisite self-care, which makes this chapter so important: 60 percent of what you use on your skin is absorbed into your body. So in order to prevent the reintroduction of the very same toxins you are working so hard to get rid of, it's time to look at the grooming products you use every day.

Take a good look at the self-care products you use for your hair and teeth; the cosmetics you use routinely; as well as the soaps, body scrubs, moisturizers, lotions and creams, and so on that you use to get clean and feel youthful and fresh. Bear in mind that your skin is permeable, so while it exudes toxins when you sweat, it also absorbs them from any you put on your skin or even use to brush your teeth.

If you have a spare moment, visit the Environmental Working Group's Skin Deep Cosmetic Database (http://www.ewg.org/skindeep) and get the lowdown on the items you are currently using. I think you'll be motivated to investigate some healthier alternatives!

One easy way to buy better-for-you cosmetics and self-care items is to shop at health food stores or retailers like Whole Foods—or you can go simple and use coconut oil for your hair and skin. Find what works for you—you don't have to go crazy with this assignment. If you want a full cleanse, try some of the great homemade self-care recipes in this chapter. They're fun, easy to make, and smell great. They will also nourish your health and looks without using harmful chemicals.

SALT DETOX BATH RECIPE

Soaking in an alkalizing liquid, one that helps pull impurities out of your skin, is a time-honored way to help your body get rid of trapped toxins and water weight, which in turn results in a smaller number on the scale and looser-fitting clothing! If you're up for it, try a nightly or every-other-night detox bath during your 7-Day Superfood Cleanse. It should be done at night because this bath makes you feel drowsy and helps you sleep, in part due to the magnesium boost from the Epsom salts. Fortunately, a detox bath is easy to do at home, with ingredients you probably already have in your kitchen or bathroom. Keep a glass of tepid water nearby to enjoy while bathing—some people get thirsty in a detox bath.

1 cup Epsom salts or baking soda (or a combination of the two)
A few drops your favorite essential oil, if desired (I use 10 drops of bergamot oil)

1. Begin adding comfortably hot water to your bathtub. As it begins to fill, pour in the salts and/or baking soda and the essential oil.
2. Fill the bathtub to nearly full so you can fully submerge yourself.
3. Soak in the bath for 30 minutes or as long as desired.

HAIR

Once upon a time, most people rubbed oil into the dry ends of their hair, washed their tresses with the same soap they used on their body, and then gave their hair a quick rinse with lemon juice, apple cider vinegar, or beer to help create shine and make locks easier to comb. Today, things are a whole lot more chemical-heavy, due to a staggering array of hair-care cleansers, conditioners, and other treatments that contain laboratory-created ingredients with names like aminophenol, diaminobenzene, phenylenediamine, phthalates, parabens, and xylene. These chemicals are absorbed by the body and can lead to fluid buildup, sluggishness, chemical sensitivities, foggy thinking, sleep abnormalities, and lowered immune system function—many of the same conditions you are trying to remedy with the 7-Day Superfood Cleanse! So during these seven days, use chemical-free hair-care and other grooming products. You may be pleasantly surprised by how great you look and feel when you stick with nature-made ingredients.

BANANA PRE-CONDITIONER
MAKES ABOUT ⅓ CUP

Banana and coconut team up to create a terrific pre-shampoo conditioner. Bananas are rich in tryptophan, an essential amino acid that strengthens hair, as well as potassium, a mineral that helps make your hair shine. Coconut moisturizes and nourishes your hair and scalp. This conditioner is great for all types of hair and works especially well on tresses that have been damaged by sun, chlorine, chemicals, or heat styling. You'll need a shower cap or plastic wrap for this one.

> 1 medium banana
> 1 tablespoon liquid coconut oil, almond oil, extra-virgin olive oil,
>   or another favorite oil

1. Using a food processor or blender, process the ingredients into a thick paste. Add ½ tablespoon of water or coconut milk if the mixture seems too thick. Add a few teaspoons of coconut flour if the mixture seems too thin.
2. Apply the treatment to dry hair, separating tresses to coat all strands.
3. Tuck your hair into a shower cap and allow the conditioner to penetrate hair for 30 minutes or more.
4. Shampoo and condition your hair as usual.

TOTALLY COCONUT PRE-SHAMPOO HAIR MASK

MAKES 1½ CUPS (ONE TREATMENT)

This coconut milk–based conditioning treatment is whipped up from things you probably already have in your kitchen: coconut milk (homemade or canned), an avocado, and some coconut oil. These superfood ingredients nourish the hair and scalp and leave strands super soft and shiny. This formula is best for normal to dry hair—it may be too moisturizing for oilier tresses.

1 avocado, peeled and pitted
1 cup coconut milk
2 tablespoons liquid coconut oil, almond oil, extra-virgin olive oil, or another favorite oil

1. Place the avocado in a food processor and pulse until mashed. (You can also mash the avocado in a bowl with a fork.)
2. Add the coconut milk and coconut oil to the avocado. Pulse until blended.
3. Apply to dry hair. Cover with a plastic shower cap, if desired.
4. Allow the mixture to penetrate hair for 15 minutes or longer.
5. Shampoo thoroughly with warm water to remove the mixture.

SEMI-HOMEMADE SHAMPOO
MAKES A LITTLE MORE THAN ½ CUP

Soothing, softening, moisturizing coconut milk shampoo nourishes your scalp and each strand of your hair. Note that it requires some commercial shampoo, however. If you don't have any baby shampoo on hand, go ahead and use whatever shampoo you have.

¼ cup coconut milk (homemade or canned)
⅓ cup organic baby shampoo or baby wash
1 teaspoon olive oil or almond oil
10 drops of your favorite essential oil (optional)

1. Combine all ingredients in a bottle or jar and shake vigorously until combined. Store in the refrigerator until ready to use.
2. To use, apply 1 or 2 tablespoons to the roots of your hair and massage into your scalp. There won't be a ton of lather, but your hair will get clean and be baby soft!
3. Rinse. If desired, follow up with your favorite conditioner.

COCONUT DETANGLER
MAKES ABOUT 1 CUP

I have thick, wavy, dry hair that can be difficult to manage. When I was growing up, my mother went through huge quantities of No Tears Detangler as she tried to tame my mane. Coconut Detangler is a more natural version of the commercial formula. You can find vegetable glycerin and grapefruit seed extract at just about any health food store.

8 ounces distilled water
1 teaspoon aloe vera gel
½ teaspoon coconut oil
10–15 drops grapefruit seed extract
1–2 drops vegetable glycerin
1–2 drops essential oil

1. Fill a spray bottle with the ingredients and shake like mad.
2. Spray on wet or dry tangled hair, or mist hair after shampooing to use as a light leave-in conditioner.

FACE

I think it's safe to say that each of us would like a glowing, clear complexion. I'm here to tell you that you can have just that, without resorting to any of the questionable ingredients many commercial skincare products use. Commercial nature-based complexion care products are great to use during the 7-Day Superfood Cleanse, but they aren't your only option: You can also choose to make your own skincare products using these fun, easy, economical, and beautifying recipes!

ANTI-ACNE MASK
MAKES ONE APPLICATION

The small amount of turmeric and coconut oil in this recipe help kill the bacteria that create breakouts, while treating the inflammation that makes skin look blotchy. In addition, banana refreshes and softens the skin, making this a terrific all-purpose mask.

½ ripe banana
1 tablespoon liquid coconut oil
¼ teaspoon turmeric powder

1. In a bowl, mash the banana into a smooth paste.
2. Mix in the coconut oil and turmeric, stirring until smooth and thoroughly combined.
3. Apply a thick coat of the mixture onto clean skin, covering face, neck, and décolletage.
4. Massage the mixture in circular motions.
5. Allow mixture to penetrate the skin for 15 minutes.
6. Remove with a soft cloth and cool water.

AVOCADO COCONUT MASK

MAKES ONE APPLICATION

I love facial masks. When I was a teenager, I would give myself a facial every Saturday. When I got older and moved to Manhattan, I would get a professional facial each week. Today, though I am still living in Manhattan, I no longer have time for professional facial treatments, so I've gone back to the homemade facials of my youth. This one is a particular favorite. It leaves skin soft, supple, and healthy thanks to the skin-nourishing fats in avocado and coconut.

¼ ripe avocado
1 tablespoon liquid coconut oil
½ teaspoon nutmeg, preferably freshly grated

1. In a bowl, mash the avocado into a smooth paste.
2. Mix in coconut oil and nutmeg, stirring until smooth and thoroughly combined.
3. Apply a thick coat of the mixture to clean skin, covering face, neck, and décolletage.
4. Massage the mixture in circular motions.
5. Allow the mixture to penetrate the skin for 15 minutes.
6. Remove with a soft cloth and cool water.

BRIGHTENING MASK
MAKES ONE APPLICATION

Lemon is a natural exfoliator and astringent that helps slough off dull, dead skin cells and makes pores appear smaller. Honey softens the skin, and coconut protects.

> 1 tablespoon raw honey
> 1 tablespoon liquid coconut oil
> ½ tablespoon lemon juice
> 2 teaspoons (or more) lemon zest

1. In a small bowl, whisk together all ingredients until completely combined.
2. Apply a thick coat to clean skin, covering face, neck, and décolletage.
3. Massage the mixture in circular motions.
4. Allow the mixture to penetrate the skin for 15 minutes.
5. Remove with a soft cloth and cool water.

WHIPPED COCONUT MOISTURIZER
MAKES ABOUT ⅓ CUP

I love this recipe. It's so luxurious, and easy and fun to make. It also makes an impressive gift! You'll need a stand mixer with a whisk attachment (or a hand mixer) to make this moisturizer, as well as a small, sealable jar in which to keep it. (You can buy small jars at any pharmacy—in the aisle where travel-sized toiletries are sold—or a craft store.)

> ¼ cup coconut oil
> 5 drops your favorite essential oil

1. In the bowl of a mixer, using the whisk attachment, whip the coconut oil until it's light and fluffy.
2. While the mixer running, add the essential oil
3. Scrape the moisturizer into a cosmetic jar (or jars) and keep it in a cool, dark place.

HANDS AND BODY

Self-care products can contain a large number of ingredients that may affect your health. These ingredients include parabens, preservatives that mimic estrogen and encourage the growth of cancerous tumors; sodium lauryl sulfate, a lathering agent that irritates skin; the preservative benzyl alcohol, which can burn skin and lower immune system function; and dozens more. One of the easiest ways to avoid these dangerous—and detox-stopping—ingredients is to go natural and opt for store-bought or homemade ingredients based on whole, unprocessed plant compounds. If you need a few recipes for these, keep reading. Here are a few cleanse-friendly products designed to help you detoxify while helping your skin look and feel beautiful.

NOURISHING BODY WASH
MAKES ABOUT 1¼ CUPS

This nourishing body wash provides a lovely natural alternative to commercial body washes. Feel free to customize it any way you like! Vegetable glycerin, the secret to suds, creates heaps of bubbles and can be purchased at health food stores and craft supply stores. You'll need a squeeze bottle for this body wash. You can also pour it into a tubful of warm water and use it as bubble bath. (My kids love it!)

½ cup coconut milk
⅔ cup unscented liquid castile soap
3 teaspoons liquid coconut oil, almond oil, extra-virgin olive oil,
   or another favorite oil
5 drops of your favorite essential oil
2 teaspoons vegetable glycerin

1. Add all ingredients to a clean, empty squeeze bottle and shake vigorously to blend.
2. Shake before each use.

BATH FIZZIES

MAKES 1–3 DOZEN, DEPENDING ON SIZE

Bath bombs are all the rage these days. Drop one into the bath and watch it fizz as it infuses the water with lovely scents and skincare benefits. If you make your own, you control what goes into them.

You can get citric acid (a citrus-derived vitamin C powder, sometimes called sour salt), at a health food store, a craft store, or a shop that sells candy-making supplies. You'll also need some molds for the fizzies, but they're easy to find wherever soap-making supplies are sold, or you can use a mini muffin tin to make these great little bath bombs.

1 cup baking soda
½ cup citric acid
½ cup cornstarch
2 tablespoons Epsom salts
2 tablespoons coconut oil, almond oil, extra-virgin olive oil, or another favorite oil
5–6 teaspoons coconut water
5–10 few drops of your favorite essential oil (optional)

1. In a large bowl, whisk together the baking soda, citric acid, cornstarch, and Epsom salts.

2. Pour the coconut oil into the mixture and work in with a dough cutter, continuing until the mixture resembles sand.

3. In a separate bowl, whisk together the coconut water and essential oils.

4. Stir the liquid mixture into the powder mixture 1 teaspoon at a time. The mixture will foam slightly with each addition—this is normal.

5. Continue to stir in liquid, 1 teaspoon at a time, until the mixture resembles slightly damp sand. (You want it to be dry, but with just enough moisture that when you squeeze a handful together, it sticks together in a lump.)

6. Once the mixture is ready, press it firmly and tightly into each mold. You do not need to prepare the molds in any way.

7. Allow the mixture to dry for a minimum of 4 hours, or overnight.

8. Remove the bath bombs from the molds and store in an airtight container until ready to use.

BEACH BODY POLISH RECIPE

MAKES 1 CUP

I love body scrubs. This lovely homemade version of body polish is made with salts that will invigorate your skin and give it a gorgeous glow. Scraped into a pretty glass jar, it makes a wonderful gift.

½ cup liquid coconut oil, almond oil, extra-virgin olive oil,
   or another favorite oil
10 drops of your favorite essential oil or oils
¼ cup sea salt
¼ cup Epsom salts

1. In a large bowl, whisk together the coconut oil and essential oil.
2. Add the sea salt and Epsom salts and stir until thoroughly combined.
3. Put the mixture into a sealable container and keep in a cool, dry place.

WHIPPED BODY BUTTER

MAKES ONE CUP

This whipped moisturizer is great for keeping skin healthy, moisturized, and blemish-free. It can be used on the face as well as the body.

½ cup shea butter
¼ cup coconut oil
¼ cup jojoba oil
5–10 drops favorite essential oil or oils

1. In a double boiler, melt together the shea butter, coconut oil, and jojoba oil, stirring until smooth.
2. Remove from the heat and stir in the essential oil.
3. Scrape the mixture into the bowl of a stand mixer and place in the refrigerator for 20 minutes or more, until the oils fully harden.
4. Return the bowl to the stand mixer and, using the whisk attachment, whip the mixture until fluffy, with the consistency of frosting.
5. Put the mixture into a sealable container and store in a cool, dry place.

HOMEMADE SUGAR SCRUB

MAKES ABOUT ¾ CUP

Sugar scrubs work a lot like salt scrubs: They use natural ingredients to exfoliate, invigorate, and soften skin. This scrub has the antibacterial, antimicrobial, and humectant benefits of both honey and coconut oil, and not only helps keep skin clear of breakouts, but softens and moisturizes, as well.

1 tablespoon coconut oil, almond oil, extra-virgin olive oil,
  or another favorite oil
2 tablespoons raw honey
5 drops of your favorite essential oil
¼ cup sea salt
¼ cup organic sugar
1 tablespoon lemon juice

1. In a medium bowl, whisk together the coconut oil, honey, and essential oil. Set the mixture aside.
2. In another small bowl, blend the salt, sugar, and lemon juice until it becomes crumbly.
3. Pour the salt mixture over the honey mixture and stir until smooth.
4. Scrape the mixture into a sealable glass container.

HOMEMADE BUG REPELLENT

For a quick bug repellent, blend together 8 ounces of liquid coconut oil and 40–50 drops of geranium, lavender, patchouli, rosewood, or lemon essential oil. Apply it as a body oil to repel mosquitoes, no-see-ums, fleas, ticks, chiggers, and other pests.

HOMEMADE SUNSCREEN

MAKES 1 CUP

Sunscreen is a sticky topic in my household. I personally don't like the stuff—I don't like the way it feels or all the crazy chemicals it contains, and, living in New York, I am slightly vitamin D deficient, so I like to get as much direct sunlight as possible. Having said that, my mother's family, originally from Scotland, has been plagued by skin cancer. So I know the importance of shielding your skin from ultraviolet rays. This homemade sunscreen, while not as powerful as the stuff you can buy in a drugstore, is a welcome alternative to commercial products. Plus, if you choose to include one of the essential oils listed below, this sunscreen lotion doubles as an insect repellent. You can buy zinc oxide powder at your local pharmacy.

½ cup almond oil
¼ cup coconut oil
¼ cup grated beeswax
1 teaspoon vitamin E oil (optional, for extra moisturizing)
2 tablespoons shea butter (optional, for extra moisturizing)
2 tablespoons zinc oxide powder (this adds a natural SPF of 20+ or more to the formula)
5 drops favorite essential oil (optional; to use as a bug repellent, choose geranium, lavender, patchouli, rosewood, or lemon)

1. In a double boiler, combine all ingredients except the zinc oxide and essential oil, if using. Melt the ingredients together, stirring until thoroughly combined and smooth.
2. Remove the mixture from the heat and allow to cool slightly.
3. Stir in the zinc oxide (being very careful not to inhale any) and essential oil, if using.
4. Scrape the mixture into a sealable jar or bottle.
5. Store in a dark, cool place.

ABOVE THE NECK

I am going to sound like a broken record, but I'll say it again: Wherever and whenever you use chemical ingredients, you run the risk of absorbing them into your body, where they can have a negative impact on your ability to excrete toxins, flush out water weight, maintain a strong immune system, and stay fit and healthy. That's why I've included nature-based recipes for the self-care and cosmetic products you may use on your teeth and eyes.

HOMEMADE TOOTHPASTE WITH COCONUT OIL

MAKES ¾ CUP

Coconut has antimicrobial, antifungal, and antiviral qualities, making it the perfect ingredient for cleaning and protecting your teeth. Try this homemade toothpaste and see how wonderful coconut can be for your oral hygiene.

6 tablespoons coconut oil
6 tablespoons baking soda
1 drop peppermint oil
1 teaspoon stevia (or more if you like it sweeter)

1. In a bowl, whisk together all ingredients until the mixture has a light, almost fluffy texture.
2. Scrape the mixture into a sealable container.
3. To use, dip your toothbrush into the toothpaste and brush as you normally would. Rinse.
4. Store toothpaste in your bathroom or in the refrigerator.

COCONUT EYE CREAM
MAKES 2 10-MILLILITER COSMETIC JARS

I am an enormous fan of eye cream. Because of the enormous quantities of sun I enjoyed as a child in Australia and California, fine lines have begun to show up around my eyes. To help smooth them, I use a lot of eye cream. I keep a jar of the stuff in each bathroom at home and carry some with me in my purse. (Don't tell anyone, but I've even been known to pat on a bit while sitting in one of my children's rehearsals or at lunch with my friends.) This particular cream turns to liquid once the temperature rises above 78°F, so keep it in the fridge or a cool room.

> 2 tablespoons coconut oil
> 1 teaspoon vitamin E oil
> 1 tablespoon primrose oil
> 1 drop of your favorite essential oil (preferably nothing too strong)

1. In a double boiler over low heat, warm the coconut oil, vitamin E oil, and primrose oil. Stir until smooth and thoroughly combined.
2. Remove the mixture from the heat and let it cool slightly.
3. Stir in the essential oil.
4. Scrape the cream into a small jar or other sealable container.
5. Store in the refrigerator or other cool place.

10

COMING OFF THE DETOX

CONGRATULATIONS! YOU'VE MADE IT! Your body has just been through an incredible experience. For seven days, you've paid exquisite attention to your health, consuming foods and drinks that energize and alkalize you, help flush out toxins, and encourage weight loss. You are probably feeling cleaner, clearer, more energetic, and lighter than you have in a while. It is wonderful not to feel puffy, to lose weight, to have great skin, to glow, and to feel energetic, creative, and slim. What may not be as much fun, for some of you, is to go without your daily cup of coffee or your nightly drink, or perhaps it's bread, chips, or sweets you'll miss.

Before you dive into a bowl of ice cream, pour yourself a glass of wine, or go out for pizza, read this chapter—because just as there is a right way to ease into a cleanse, there is also a right way to come off a cleanse. Here's how to do it safely:

- Do not dive into packaged food, fast food, junk food, or factory food. These chemical-heavy foods are not only bad for your health, they contribute to bloat and weight gain. If you want to eat something, try real food. You've worked too hard over the last seven days to let a handful of Doritos take you out!
- Do not dump food into your system! You may be tempted to introduce large quantities of food to your freshly detoxed body. Please resist! Digestion takes a lot of work! Eat moderately and your body will thank you. A great rule of thumb is to not eat more than the amount of food you can fit in your palm at any one time.
- Don't overdose on animal products, wheat, sugar, alcohol, and so on. Instead of diving into all the things you gave up while detoxing, gradually add small amounts of these foods back into your daily diet (maybe ¼ cup of meat or poultry per meal, no more than twice a day for the first week post-cleanse), in order

to not experience headaches, digestive distress, bloating, moodiness, and lethargy. Go slow, slow, slow.

- Remember that you can course-correct. If you do a few foods a bit too quickly and are in gastric distress, I promise you'll be okay. You may feel uncomfortable, but you haven't permanently hurt yourself. Just take a few steps back and slow back down.
- Continue having green drinks and protein for breakfast. Forever.
- Keep consuming chia. Forever.
- Drink water. And more water. And then some more water. It will keep your body clean and allow it to efficiently flush out the toxins that can lead to water weight and bloat.
- Keep up with anything that you loved and that worked well for you during the 7-Day Superfood Cleanse. They are self-care tools that you can use forever.
- Movement. Keep moving your body, every single day. Daily movement not only keeps your metabolism healthy, muscles strong, and circulation in good order, it helps move lymph through your body, so it can collect and dispose of the toxins that can lead to puffiness, bloating, lackluster skin, and a host of other troubles.

THE COME-OFF-A-CLEANSE MENU

For those of you who like to follow menus, here is one for you. This post-cleanse menu is flexible enough for you to use for the rest of your life, if you'd like to. In fact, I suggest it! Eating this way most of the time is a great way to lose weight, maintain weight loss, and help your body stay at the top of its game.

THROUGHOUT THE DAY

- Sip water throughout the day. Feel free to add lemon or lime juice, apple cider vinegar, or cucumber slices to it. I suggest keeping water with you at all times, just so you have it handy.

- Drink a large glass of lukewarm water (not cold!) with a squirt (about 1 teaspoon) of lemon or lime juice, or a splash of apple cider vinegar, every morning before you have breakfast.

SUGGESTED BREAKFAST

- One *Green Drink* (pages 54–57)
- A combo of protein and veggie breakfast. This can be 1–2 whole eggs and veggies (such as a spinach omelet) or a salad with nuts and/or beans, veggie chili with beans, chickpea-veggie curry, bean and veggie salad or sauté, and so on.
- Alternatively, you might try some sautéed veggies and one serving of nitrite-free bacon or breakfast sausage, or even nitrite-free deli meat, some poultry, or red meat from last night's dinner.
- 1 cup of black, green, or herbal tea

SUGGESTED MID-MORNING SNACK

Choose one or two of the following:
- A cup of herbal tea (your choice) or *Lemon-Ginger Detox Drink* (page 64)
- A handful of nuts (about ¼ cup)
- Veggies with hummus or bean dip or guacamole (made without dairy) or nut butter
- A cup of gazpacho or vegetable soup
- One or more tomatoes, sliced and drizzled with extra-virgin olive oil and your vinegar of choice, and sprinkled with salt, pepper, and/or chopped herbs, if you like
- *Kale Chips* (pages 107 and 108)

LUNCH

Feel free to switch the lunch and dinner menus if it is easier for you to do that.
- One large salad (this can be as large as you'd like it—use salad greens and any veggies you like). Add ½ cup beans, ¼ cup nuts

or so, or a portion of poultry or red meat, about the size of a deck of playing cards (a bit less than one cup, chopped), for protein.

• Vinaigrette or olive oil and lemon juice dressing, made by whisking together 2 tablespoons of olive oil, ½ tablespoon lemon juice, and salt and pepper to taste

• If you are eating out, pick up a salad and choose one of the vinaigrettes, or order a veggie-over-rice dish, such as a stir-fry or curry, and eat the salad for dinner.

MID-AFTERNOON SNACK

Choose one or two, maybe a different one than you ate in the morning.

• Seltzer with lemon or lime juice
• Veggie strips with guacamole or nut butter, hummus, or bean dip, made by whirring ¼ cup of beans, a squirt of lemon juice, one garlic clove, salt and pepper, and a splash of olive oil in your food processor
• A cup of gazpacho or vegetable soup
• One or more tomatoes, sliced, and drizzled with extra-virgin olive oil and your choice of vinegar, and sprinkled with salt, pepper, and/or chopped herbs, if you like
• *Kale Chips* (pages 107 and 108)
• *Summer Watermelon Detox Smoothie* (page 61)

DINNER

Feel free to switch lunch and dinner menus, if it is easier for you to do that. The easiest way to get plant-based protein will probably be a sauté, stir-fry, curry, or soup or stew, where you can have beans and/or nuts with the veggies.

• One *Green Drink* (pages 54–57)
• A 1-cup serving of grain (brown rice, quinoa, amaranth, millet, etc.)
• One serving of protein (poultry, red meat—the size of a deck of playing cards or a computer mouse)—or 1–2 eggs, or ¼ cup nuts or ½ cup beans
• As many sautéed veggies as you like (second helpings are fine)

Choose as many as you'd like.

- A cup of herbal tea (your choice) or *Lemon-Ginger Detox Drink* (page 64)
- Veggie strips
- *Summer Watermelon Detox Smoothie* (page 61)
- A cup of vegetable soup
- One or more tomatoes, sliced, and drizzled with extra-virgin olive oil and maybe your choice of vinegar, and sprinkled with salt, pepper, and/or chopped herbs, if you like
- *Kale Chips* (pages 107 and 108)

11

EXTENDING YOUR CLEANSE

PERSONALLY, I DON'T FEEL THAT BEING on a cleanse is difficult. I know each of us is different, but I love earmarking a period of time where I focus on improving my health by eating clean, nutrient-dense food. Instead of seeing it as deprivation, I see it is as a special gift, something I do just for me.

Sometimes when I do 5-day or even a 10-day detox with my clients, I extend my own cleanse by a few days. Why? Because I don't want it to end! Because I want more weight loss, better-looking skin, increased energy, and the heightened creativity that comes with detoxing for a few additional days. You may feel the same and wonder if you can—or should—extend your cleanse for a few days.

The answer is: Well, it depends. If you are feeling strong both physically and emotionally, don't have a pre-existing health condition to worry about, and would like to keep going for a few additional days, go ahead—but first, turn to page 32 and review the menu, shopping list, and details of the Everday Cleanse Plan. Follow it for as many extra days as you like—7 days is reasonable span. If you want to throw in one extra hardcore Quick Cleanse day, take a look at page 39 and read up on the menu, lists, tips, and tricks you'll need during an extended cleanse time. Just limit yourself to one extra Quick Cleanse day. And be ready to come off your extended cleanse the moment you become fatigued.

Please continue to get enough sleep during your extended cleanse. Flushing toxins doesn't really require you to actively do anything, but it does call for an expenditure of energy, which means you may feel a bit tired. Or you may not feel tired at all—you may feel positively giddy and energetic! Your body flushes toxins (and sends trapped water weight into your excretory system) while you sleep. So regardless of how energetic you feel, your body needs sleep to do its deepest detox work. So don't skimp. Don't burn the proverbial candle at both ends while detoxing.

One final piece of advice: Don't forget to move! Go for a walk, ski, swim, or do anything else that is going to encourage your body to sweat (a great way to detoxify) and boost your circulation—which, in turn, will encourage lymph to circulate through your body, trapping toxins and escorting them out of the body through your urine.

Often, the very thing we need to keep us looking and feeling healthy isn't anything that we actually put into our bodies—not even a superfood—it's a mindset and making a commitment.

12

POP-UP CLEANSES

MANY OF THE THINGS YOU'VE LEARNED while doing the 7-Day Superfood Cleanse, from making nutrient-dense vegan meals and green drinks to proper breathing and self-care (body brushing, for example), can be used afterward, for as long as you like. Keep these clean habits in your everyday life, and you'll continue to feel as great as you do now.

But I'm a realist: I know that many of you will go back to the foods you worked so hard to eliminate during the cleanse—coffee, cheese, bacon, pasta, bread, and so on. There is nothing wrong with this, although you will probably see the return of some bloating. Much of the puffiness will be water weight, since so many of the foods you eliminate during a cleanse encourage the body to hold on to excess water. But I need to be straight with you: Some of what you think is bloat may be fat, pure and simple.

REBOOTING THE CLEANSE

If you've begun to put on a bit of water weight and bloat, there *is* a solution: A reboot with a pop-up cleanse. Check your calendar, clear off 1–3 days, and turn to page 32, where you'll find the shopping list, menu,

---

WHEN ONE THING IS TO BLAME
FOR YOUR BLOAT

If you find yourself returning to pre-detox levels of puffiness after doing the 7-Day Superfood Cleanse, stop for a minute and ask yourself what's to blame. Is it the 9 p.m. dinners? The nightly glasses of wine? All that Greek yogurt? Whatever the cause of your bloat, removing it could be enough to get you back into your skinny jeans and leave you feeling energetic.

and instructions for the Everyday Cleanse Plan. You can create a short detox for yourself—enough to lose a bit of fat and 3 pounds or so in water weight. The Everyday Cleanse Plan is safe enough to use for a weekly pop-up cleanse, a monthly pop-up cleanse, or once a season, as needed.

This is important: I also want you to do some type of sweaty exercise while you're detoxing. If you're a walker, you can have your walk, but I also want you to work up a sweat and perspire out the water weight that is bloating your belly and face. Sweaty exercise will keep your metabolism strong, too.

THE EXTREME POP-UP MINI-CLEANSE

There's another option to a 2- or 3-day pop-up cleanse that is faster, deeper, and more restrictive: a 1-day cleanse following the Quick Cleanse Plan. On page 39, you'll find the shopping list, menu, and instructions for this accelerated weight- and water-loss plan. Please limit yourself to a single day, however, because the Quick Cleanse Plan, which is mostly liquid, is too restrictive to do for more than a day at a time. But it's perfect to use before a special event to ensure that you look the way you want to look in your little black dress, or if you want a dramatic jump-start to a weight loss program. If you're healthy, with no pre-existing health conditions, you can do a 1-day pop-up cleanse using the Fast Cleanse Plan as often as once a week, although you may find it easier to dive into the plan once every two to four weeks.

Some sort of sweaty exercise is just as important to do while on the Extreme Pop-Up Mini-Cleanse as it is on the Everyday Cleanse Plan. Again, if you're a walker, you can have your walk, but I also want you to sweat—it'll help you lose the water weight that bloats your belly and face, and it'll keep your metabolism strong. Get moving!

13

TROUBLESHOOTING

W HENEVER YOU EMBARK ON SOMETHING NEW, you're bound to run into a thing or two that you weren't expecting—and that can cause more than a little worry. When this happens, it's important to have help from someone who can walk you through your concerns—especially when they involve your health!

Although I can't be with you in person, I have an idea of the kinds of glitches you may experience. In the hundreds of times I've run detoxes, certain matters come up again and again. This is the section where I shine some light on them and walk you through how to handle them.

HEALTH CONCERNS

- **You have a health condition/food allergy/intolerance/aversion and can't (or don't want to) eat an ingredient I call for in one (or more) of my recipes.** Don't eat it! You can omit it entirely or substitute another ingredient. If red beans make you gassy, use mung beans. If your doctor has told you to avoid raw kale, use romaine lettuce. The 7-Day Superfood Cleanse works because it is flexible!
- **Your mom and best friend say that cleanses are dangerous, and now you're worried about diving in.** Get each of them a copy of *The 7-Day Superfood Cleanse* and invite them to join you! This is a whole-food and drink detox that uses superfoods and other nourishing ingredients to help you ditch the bloat, release water weight, lose pounds, squash cravings, and reset your eating habits. It is not about deprivation, surviving on weird drinks, eating a limited number of foods for long periods, or taking supplements.
- **You are now peeing more.** Good!
- **A lot more!** Good! Seriously, it is all good. That trapped water needs to leave your body somehow, right? Urinating is the fastest

way to get large amounts of trapped water out of your body, thus eliminating bloat and flushing toxins.

• **You are constipated.** There is more fiber in the 7-Day Superfood Cleanse than you may have been consuming in your everyday life. Give yourself two or three days and you should be on a more regular schedule. To ensure your comfort—and your regularity—be sure to drink eight glasses of water a day and fit in some daily exercise. Even gentle movement, like walking, counts! These all help the body eliminate more easily.

• **Or you are in the bathroom more frequently.** For some people, the larger amount of veggies they are eating can cause looser and/ or more frequent bowel movements. This, too, is normal. If this is you, suss out if there is a specific food you are eating that is causing you to go more often. You can do this by thinking back to the last thing you ate. If you do this enough, you'll eventually track down the particular ingredient that is causing you trouble. Your job then is to cut back on that ingredient or remove it altogether, and replace it with another ingredient. If there isn't a single culprit, make sure you're eating some grains (such as brown or red or black rice or millet) with lunch, to help bind what you're eating, and keep up your water intake. Most people experience this shock to the digestive system for only a couple of days.

• **Your sense of smell (or hearing or touch) is heightened.** Weird, right? This is actually one of my favorite side effects of detoxing. There is no scientific explanation for this (sorry!), but you may notice it. Here's my theory: Certain foods either depress or stimulate our central nervous system. The limbic system, which is where our sense of smell originates, is a part of the central nervous system. When you eat foods that artificially suppress or excite your nervous system, your senses are compromised and they can't perceive things as they actually are. Once you remove these foods, you suddenly sense things just as they are. You may feel more sensitive, but in truth, your senses are simply working without the filter—or rather, the fog—caused by certain foods.

- **You aren't losing huge amounts of weight.** One of the most interesting things I've seen my clients do is personalize a program to fit in some of their favorite, hard-to-give-up foods—Greek yogurt, for example, or chocolate, coffee, wine, or fruit. If you haven't completely put these foods away for the entirety of the detox, you may find that the results of your weight loss efforts aren't what you want them to be. This also applies to late night eaters. Dining early, eating light, and staying away from post-supper snacking is a real struggle for many people—but if you can stick with the program, your weight-loss efforts will pay off.
- **You feel irritable.** When we come off certain addictive foods, certain feelings may come up. Some of these are emotional, such as loss or longing. Others are biochemical. Your body gets used to having certain ingredients around and begins to feel jittery and moody without them. (Coffee and sugar, I am looking at you!) If this is something you're experiencing, go grab some herbal tea or a glass of water with lemon juice. Drink it down and go outside for a walk. The water, the movement, and the air on your skin will calm you and bring you back to center. Irritability won't last for more than a couple of days, if that.
- **You have a headache.** When we remove addictive substances from our diet we often feel headachy, as our bodies get used to living without a food that may have altered the way our central nervous system does its job. Coming off of alcohol, coffee, sugar, and wheat, in particular can leave you feeling headachy. Pour yourself a large glass of water with lemon and drink up. If you can get yourself outside for a walk in the fresh air, please do. The fresh air wakes you up, while the movement encourages blood flow to the brain.
- **You are hungry!** Not a problem! Just eat bigger portions of the prescribed food in the 7-Day Superfood Cleanse and be sure to include the suggested snacks in your daily meal plan.
- **You are full!!** A lot of people report that the 7-Day Superfood Cleanse actually leaves them feeling full. This is kind of exciting, when you consider the reputation cleanses have for leaving people

ravenously hungry. If you are full, don't feel compelled to finish a meal, and go ahead and skip the snack.

- **You feel tired.** This isn't one that most detoxers experience. Still, it does come up for some people. Detoxing is hard work. Your body is laboring to remove toxins from the body, which can be exhausting! In addition, you aren't eating the animal protein that you may be used to. Bump up your bedtime by an hour and sleep in, if you can. In one or two days you will find your energy levels not just returning, but soaring.

- **You feel cold.** Are you doing this detox during cold weather? If you are eating a lot of salads and other uncooked foods when the temperature outside is cool, you may feel a bit chilly. This is completely normal. To keep yourself warm, opt for soup over salad, enjoy plenty of hot herbal tea, and use plenty of warming spices, such as cumin, ginger, cinnamon, curry, turmeric, garlic, and hot sauce.

LIFE CONCERNS

- **You live with someone who makes it hard for you to stay healthy.** I know all about this one and sympathize with you! In my case, that *someone* is my husband. He likes wine, as much as I do—and he will not stop bringing it into the house just because I am on a cleanse. What I do is admit to him that I find it hard to resist the vino, but, being the intrepid soul that I am, I will indeed resist the vino. Then I ask him to make sure I resist the vino! Asking for someone's help to keep you on track may work beautifully, but if the person is a saboteur, you'll need a different strategy: Don't tell him or her you are on a cleanse and you'll avoid awakening their inner troublemaker. If you are offered something that won't support your goals, simply raise your glass of seltzer and lime and say, "Skoal!" (That's Danish for "No thanks! I'm all set here with my water!")

- **You have a dinner party (or other event) coming up.** This is another one I know well! Don't give up on a social event just because you're on a cleanse—there's no need! Simply eat the foods that are detox-healthy and leave the rest. It can help to have a green juice or a glass of tomato juice or *Chia Fresca* (page 100) before you leave the house so you'll be full. This will ensure that you lead with your desire to be social instead of with your tummy. That is a powerful, often underrated tip for staying on any food plan.

- **You are traveling.** If you have a chance, get online and do a search of every airport, airline, restaurant, and hotel you'll be passing through on your trip. You can easily plan ahead: Pack a few bottled green juices, if you'd like to be safe, and, if you have to, jump onto a green juice site and arrange for a half dozen or more bottles to be delivered to your hotel room. If green drinks are absolutely undoable, have a salad for breakfast (see page 74 for more information about this).

- **You have an almost uncontrollable desire to throw away everything in your home.** Isn't that an awesome feeling? As we work internally to get rid of certain foods, toxins, and weight, we want to declutter our external world as well. It's only natural! Most people on a cleanse experience a strong desire to start tossing things away, usually around day 5. I say go with it and get some cleaning done! It is a powerful impulse—and one that you can give in to for the good of everyone around you! (Who doesn't like a spotless, organized home?)

- **You have done one day of the Quick Cleanse Plan and don't want to do the second day.** Then don't do it. You can do the Everyday Cleanse Plan instead.

- **You love the Quick Cleanse Plan and want to do it for several days in a row.** If two non-consecutive days are great, several days of the Quick Cleanse Plan in a row must be great, right? Well . . . no. I completely understand the desire to dive in and move quickly, but the Quick Cleanse Plan doesn't have a lot of calories, and it is very liquid heavy. Not that those are bad things, but it'll be safer if you limit it to days 4 and 6, and then maybe add an extra Quick Cleanse day at the end of your 7-Day Superfood Cleanse.

- **You don't want to exercise.** I know. I don't want to exercise, either. I do love to walk, though, and few things feel better to me than a morning run on a misty day. But I admit that I refuse to go into a gym, and I really couldn't care less about team sports. My point? Find something that you enjoy enough to not want to put it off. And do it daily. I seriously do not care what it is, whether it's cycling or dancing around the living room or going to a fitness class. Just do it.

SHOPPING, COOKING, AND MEAL PREP

- **You are on a limited budget.** There are a few things you can do to keep costs down while doing the 7-Day Superfood Cleanse:
  - **Make all food and drinks yourself.** This is probably the greatest cost-saving measure of all.
  - **Buy less expensive ingredients.** You'll find that many of the recipes in this book give you plenty of options. If arugula is too pricey, substitute romaine. If kale is overpriced at your neighborhood market, pick up cabbage instead.
  - **Go with produce that is less expensive than organic.** I know, I know—one of the reasons to do a detox is to shed toxins. Couldn't using regular (non-organic) produce mean adding in toxins as fast as you're removing them? In an ideal world, everyone would use all-organic ingredients, but I'm a realist. You won't shed quite as many toxins, it's true, if you use "regular" produce, but you'll get plenty of other benefits nonetheless, such as better control over carb cravings, less bloat, and more weight loss.
- **You don't cook.** That's fine. Throughout the book there are plenty of tips on how to use premade food and green drinks from delis, health food stores, and restaurants. You will be just fine (though I do challenge you to do a bit of cooking).
- **You don't have a blender or juicer and have no plans to buy either one.** That's fine, too. As much as I want you to try making your own green drinks, I know that not everyone is down with

that. Go ahead and purchase your daily drink from a health food store, juice joint, or even supermarket. You'll find plenty of suggestions on how to do this (and what to choose) in this book.

- **You don't have time to make your own lunches and/or dinners.** This is also fine! You are welcome to pick up your lunches and dinners from places that offer takeout food, such as healthy salad bars, supermarkets, and restaurants—as long as detox-friendly options are on the menu. If your challenge is that you don't have time to cook but really would like to make your own meals, here are some ideas:

    - **Make large batches of quinoa, brown or another rice, millet, beans, and soups on the weekend** before you start the 7-Day Superfood Cleanse and freeze them for use during the week.
    - **Make double batches of dishes at night,** so you have food to enjoy for several days.
    - **Hire a friend or even a local cooking school student to make your meals** for you and package them for quick grab-and-go eating.

EATING

- **You can't live without meat. Or Greek yogurt. Or cheese. Or coffee. Or your nightly glass of wine. Or whatever.** Seven days. I bet you can do it for 7 days. Once the 7 days are over, you are welcome to go back to any of the foods you've given up for the week. I think you'll feel so great that you won't go back to everything you once ate—but if you want to, you won't hurt my feelings a single bit!
- **You are not a morning person and the thought of putting anything in your body before noon makes you queasy.** Please drink a glass of room temperature water with lemon or apple cider vinegar within 20 minutes of waking. If you need a bit of time to handle the green drink, go ahead and give up your mid-morning snack and have your green drink then.

- **Vegetables for breakfast? Really?** Yes! Isn't it exciting? I grew up eating veggies for breakfast. In Australia, a broiled tomato is a necessary breakfast food! (And yes, I often wake up craving tomatoes.) Around the world, most people *do* eat vegetables for breakfast, often in the form of leftovers from the previous night. I encourage you to use these 7 days to change your ideas about what you eat and when you eat, and try some new foods and new ways (and times) to enjoy them. Eating veggies (especially green ones) is alkalizing and keeps you free of cravings, while supporting more detoxing and bloat busting. Try it! I guarantee you'll feel more energetic, lighter, and focused.

- **You are craving coffee or cookies or cheese puffs or something else that isn't on the 7-Day Superfood Cleanse menu.** Oh, that's rough. And it's pretty common, too. It's hard, from both an emotional and a biochemical standpoint, to go without the foods you eat every day. What I've discovered is that green drinks really help squash those maddening cravings for junk food, carbs, sweets—or whatever your particular "poison" happens to be. Have an extra green drink instead, whenever severe cravings hit, and I'll bet they'll be gone by the time your glass is empty. If you don't have a green drink handy, herbal tea or a tomato-based vegetable drink will work almost as well.

- **You fell off the plan and had a beer.** Or a brownie. Or a yogurt. Okay. Thanks for 'fessing up. Now I am going to ask you to get back on the detox horse and start riding again. Course correction is the surest way to guarantee success.

- **You hate not eating what the rest of your family is eating.** Then serve your family what you're eating! I bet they'd love some of the soups, salads, snacks, and other recipes. You may want to supplement their dinners, but at least all of you will be eating some of the same foods.

14

DETOX FAQS

I LOVE FAQS. ASKING QUESTIONS IS HOW we learn. Lucky for me, people have a lot of questions about cleanses, from what a cleanse is to why you should try a detox to what you should eat while you're on a cleanse.

I am so excited to lend my support as you detox your body, emotions, and life and to go through a detox with you. I will enjoy being in the thick of it with you.

If you're new to detoxing—or new to me—I bet you have a few questions. I hope I've answered most of them here.

Q. Can't I just go to the health food store and buy a boxed cleanse or a supply of pressed juice from a juice press?
A. Sure you could! However, if you want to detox your body safely and easily, with no jitters or digestive upsets, it pays to learn the hows and whys of detoxing. Drinking a lot of premade green juice is one thing, but learning how to chose and even create foods and drinks that make you feel better (and find out why they make you feel better) is a priceless education. Once you know how to use food to improve your health, you can begin to create daily habits that will support your ongoing health. And should you fall off the healthy eating wagon, you can always return to the 7-Day Superfood Cleanse.

Q. Does the 7-Day Superfood Cleanse require that I survive on only juice for 7 days?
A. No! You will be eating (and drinking) in a lighter, more alkaline, less toxic, less chemicalized, and more detoxifying way for 7 days.

Q. Will I be following the same menu every day during the 7-Day Superfood Cleanse?
A. You can if you'd like to. The 7-Day Superfood Cleanse features two

menus: The Everyday Cleanse Menu, which can be followed each of the 7 days, and the Quick Cleanse Menu, which is designed to be used on days 4 and 6, if you'd like to kick things up a notch.

Q. Why can't I have coffee on the 7-Day Superfood Cleanse?

A. Coffee causes water retention and bloating—the very things we're trying to target with the 7-Day Superfood Cleanse. In addition, studies have shown that coffee raises blood glucose levels, which in turn can cause fierce cravings for sweet, carby foods (chocolate chip cookies, anyone?)—not the kind of cravings you want to be battling while on a cleanse.

Q. Why can't I have sugar on the 7-Day Superfood Cleanse?

A. Sugar is one of the most addictive substances on the planet (seriously), which is why we eat so much of it. Did you know the average American consumes the equivalent of 19 teaspoons of sugar a day? It is recommended that we consume no more than 6 teaspoons a day, if we eat any at all. Sugar causes large fluctuations in blood sugar levels, creates bloat, and can lower immune system function, lead to diabetes, damage your teeth's enamel, cause weight gain, overstimulate the nervous system (causing moodiness, aggression, hyperactivity, brain fog, and lowered mental acuity), and create powerful biochemical changes in the body that in turn make you crave (yes, you guessed it) even more sugar. Plus, your body has a hard time letting go of trapped toxins and water weight when it is filled with sugar.

Q. Why can't I have eggs on the 7-Day Superfood Cleanse?

A. Many of the foods that are removed during a cleanse *do* have health benefits. Eggs are one of them. Although they are rich in protein and omega-3 fatty acids, vitamin E, choline, selenium, biotin, vitamin B12, vitamin B2, and protein, eggs can create an acidic environment in the body, which makes it difficult to shed toxins.

Q. Why can't I have poultry, red meat, and seafood while I'm on the 7-Day Superfood Cleanse?
A. Like eggs, meat offers myriad health benefits, including B vitamins and protein. But it, too, can create an acidic environment in the body that makes it difficult to flush toxins and trapped water.

Q. Why can't I have milk products on the 7-Day Superfood Cleanse?
A. Dairy products made from cow's milk, goat's milk, sheep's milk, or any other living animal's milk— including cheese and Greek yogurt— cause bloating, encourage the body to retain water, and create an acidic environment that prevents efficient detoxing.

Q. Why can't I have alcohol on the 7-Day Superfood Cleanse?
A. Alcohol is an important part of many of our lives. We may consume it socially, either nightly or several times a week; it may be de rigueur at dinner; and we may even use it as a medication, to self-soothe after a frustrating, emotional, or overly busy day. During the 7-Day Superfood Cleanse, however, take a break from alcohol and its effects on the body, which may include damaging the heart, making it difficult for the liver to filter toxins, causing the pancreas to produce toxic substances that can lead to pancreatitis, increasing your risk of cancer, weakening your immune system, impairing brain function, changing your blood's glucose levels, weakening your resolve to make healthy choices, and lowering your inhibitions, which can in turn lead to making choices you would otherwise avoid. Alcohol also leads to carb cravings and water retention, and creates an acidic environment in the body.

Q. Why can't I have wheat and products containing gluten while on the 7-Day Superfood Cleanse?
A. Have your heard of the term *wheat belly*? It refers to the midsection bloating that results from eating gluten on a regular basis. During a cleanse, gluten is removed from your diet to help you get rid of that puffiness and head off the carb cravings that gluten can cause.

Q. Where's the fruit? I thought fruit was good for me, but I notice you don't include fruit in the 7-Day Superfood Cleanse.

A. I love fruit. It tastes amazing, and it's filled with fiber, vitamins, and all kinds of wonderful phytonutrients. But fruit also contains a good amount of sugar—natural sugar, but sugar nonetheless. Fruit is removed from the 7-Day Superfood Cleanse, not because it isn't good for you, but because it makes it hard to detoxify your body and keep cravings at bay. But luckily for you, you can load up on veggies to ensure that you are getting all the deeply nourishing produce your body needs to stay its healthiest.

Q. Why are all processed foods removed from the 7-Day Superfood Cleanse?

A. Once upon a time, when saber-toothed tigers roamed the world, humans were forced to eat what they foraged or hunted. There was no pasta, no boil-in-a-bag rice mixes, and no dried, canned, bottled, or reconstituted anything. The only food that was available was whole food, which we ate out of necessity—and which rewarded us with energy, good health, and fit bodies. When we start tampering with ingredients, however—removing this, changing the form of that, and adding chemicals here and there—we don't receive all the benefits of whole foods that nature intended. You will find it easier to lose weight, bloating, and puffiness—without energy-draining cravings—when you stick to whole foods.

Q. Why do you ask people to have a green drink in the morning?

A. Because green drinks are magical! In the world of psychology there is a belief that if you start your day feeling a specific way, you tend to carry that feeling—and the motivation that comes with it—throughout the day. When you enjoy a green drink first thing in the morning, you are also alkalizing yourself and creating a high-energy feeling that squashes cravings and leaves you feeling focused, strong, and craving-free all day. Start your day with a green drink, and you will be much less likely to reach for a muffin at 10:00 a.m. than you would if you started your day with breakfast cereal, waffles, or a bagel. If you don't believe me, just try it my way for 7 days and see how your life changes!

Q. What do you mean by "being alkaline"?

A. Alkalinity is the most efficient, healthiest place for you to be, where all of your bodily functions—including metabolism and your body's detoxification pathways—operate at their best. Do you remember learning about acid and alkaline balances back in high school chemistry? The human body's ideal pH is slightly alkaline—7.30–7.45. This is the sweet spot, the environment where the body's metabolic, enzymatic, immunologic, and repair mechanisms function most efficiently, cravings are low, energy is high, sleep is good, mental acuity is strong, and so on. If the body veers into territory that's too acidic (anything below a 7 on the pH scale), it tries to create a protective buffer to neutralize the acids. It creates this barrier by stealing alkaline minerals (such as potassium, sodium, magnesium, and calcium) from your vital organs, teeth, and bones. The results of being acidic can be fatigue, high blood pressure, kidney stones, poor immune system function, premature aging, osteoporosis, joint pain, muscle aches, mood swings, lack of focus, slow digestion and elimination, bloating, skin conditions, yeast infections, fungal infections, obesity, slow metabolism, and the inability to lose weight.

Q. Why do you ask people to drink so much water on the 7-Day Superfood Cleanse?

A. Your body is composed of about 60 percent water, which helps with digestion, nutrient absorption, blood circulation, creation of saliva, transportation of nutrients, and maintenance of body temperature. Water also helps muscles stay moist and strong, and it helps maintain brain and proper bowel function, which is particularly helpful to detoxing, because it encourages your kidneys to filter toxins out of your body through your urine. Water also creates a feeling of satiety that keeps emotional and boredom-based eating in check.

Q. Why do you restrict nighttime eating on the 7-Day Superfood Cleanse? Why does it matter when I eat something?

A. Not everyone agrees with this, but in some wellness traditions, such as traditional Chinese medicine and Ayurveda, eating late in the day is frowned on. Your body systems are slowing down so you can get a good night's sleep. Filling up your body with food when your body doesn't want to do the extra work required to digest it is thought to affect the quality of your sleep and leads to conversion and storage of unassimilated foods into fat. In my own life and those of my clients, I've noticed that one of the most powerful weight loss tools around is the early dinner. The later you eat, the lighter you should eat. A powerful way to encourage weight loss is to wrap up your evening meal by 7:00 or 7:30 p.m. and keep it light (such as a salad and/or a bowl of soup).

Q. Are you going to ask me to get a colonic?

A. No! And I won't be asking you to give yourself enemas, either. I know, I know—lots of detox gurus swear by them...but I am not one of them. End of story. There are plenty of things we'll be doing to cleanse your body from the inside out (as well as cleaning up your life)—but, if you are really hankering for a colonic or enema, be my guest.

Q. I work in an office. Will I be able to do the 7-Day Superfood Cleanse?

A. Yes—and pretty easily! Thumb through the book. As you'll see, you'll be eating real foods, which you can either prepare yourself, take out from a deli, or enjoy in a restaurant. There are no weird powders or off-putting "health" bars with weird ingredients in the 7-Day Superfood Cleanse. This detox is all about real food! It is designed to give you maximum energy during the day, when you really need it. Few of us have the luxury of taking a week off just because we're detoxing.

Q. Do I need a blender or juicer to do the 7-Day Superfood Cleanse?

A. Not necessarily. If you want to make your own green drinks (either green smoothies with a blender or green juice with a juicer), then yes, you'll need a blender or juicer. But it is just as effective to have a green drink made for you at your local health food store—just go easy on the fruit and avoid any dairy or soy additives.

Q. I have been diagnosed with an emotional eating disorder. Is it okay for me to do a cleanse?

A. Unfortunately, cleanses (detoxes, fasts, reboots, or whatever else you want to call them) often attract people whose only goal is to lose large amounts of weight fast, who have an emotional attachment to deprivation, who are frightened to consume calories, or who have a disordered relationship with food. If this applies to you, you will not be well served by a detox, since it can greatly exacerbate emotional and disordered eating.

Q. Can someone who is pregnant or breast-feeding do a cleanse?

A. If you are pregnant or breast-feeding, I'd encourage you to wait until the baby has been born and weaned to undergo a cleanse of any kind. There is a chance that some toxins can be passed to the baby in utero or through breast milk. Enjoy your pregnancy, enjoy breastfeeding, and then, when you're done, come back and celebrate by doing the 7-Day Superfood Cleanse.

Q. I'm not terrific at following directions. Can I still do the 7-Day Superfood Cleanse?

A. If following directions is difficult for you, this may not be the program for you. Here's why: I have been detoxing myself, my family, and my clients for years. In fact, I am known for my detoxes. I cannot guarantee that you'll enjoy the complete results I want for you if you don't dive in and commit to doing the (very fun, not super-difficult) work. Do the same thing you've always done, and you'll get the same results you've always had. Do something different, get something different. It makes sense, doesn't it?

RESOURCES

PRODUCE IN BULK

www.doortodoororganics.com

If you can't shop locally, ordering online is a great option. Door-to-Door Organics allows you to purchase a veggie box, fruit box, or mixed produce box in one of four sizes. All produce comes from organic farms.

www.fruitguys.com

The Fruit Guys is an online company that sends a mix of produce, highlighting seasonal items in each region of the country.

www.localharvest.org

This comprehensive site not only allows you to buy bulk produce online, it also lets you plug in your zip code and find a comprehensive lists of the nearest farmers markets, food co-ops, you-pick farms, farm stands, community-supported agricultural programs, and more throughout the United States. Most of these are rated by visitors, making it easy to choose the option you think may serve you best.

www.nfmd.org

The National Farmers Market Directory allows you to search for the nearest farmer's market by zip code. Market addresses, times, and in some cases links help you narrow down your options.

SUPERFOODS IN BULK

www.navitasnaturals.com

Navitas Naturals calls itself "The Superfood Company." With forty-nine products, plus self-care items and books, Navitas is a superfood powerhouse of a store!

www.nutiva.com

Another great place to buy natural products in bulk, Nutiva features six different coconut products, chia, hemp in several forms, and four different red palm products. Plus it has free shipping offers.

www.sunfood.com

Sun Food offers an extraordinarily wide variety of superfoods, from chlorella to chia, spirulina to sea vegetables, plus home-care and self-care items.

JUICERS AND BLENDERS

www.amazon.com

You can get just about anything on Amazon. Moreover, Amazon's service is great and its shipping is so reasonable (often free!) that is just makes sense to order juicers, blenders, and other kitchen equipment here.

www.juicing-for-health.com

Juicing for Health is a wealth of home-juicing info, including equipment reviews, explanations of the different methods of juice extraction, recipes, buying guides, and more.

www.juicerreviewsdirect.com

This site offers loads of juicer (and blender) reviews, explains the differences in juicing methods, and even offers recipes.

www.thejuicerdirectory.com

The Juicer Directory is another juicing and green smoothie fan site, with comparisons of the different types and brands of juicers and blenders, including an online store (with great prices) and helpful articles, such as "The Best Juicer for Less Than $100."

CUPS, BOTTLES, THERMOSES, AND FOOD STORAGE

www.freshwatersystems.com
Fresh Water Systems specializes in anything having to do with clean drinking water, including the top-selling brands of stainless steel water bottles at great prices and with low-cost or free shipping.

https://www.hydroflask.com
Hydro Flask offers stylish stainless steel flasks and thermoses coated in rubber, making it easy to tote your detox drinks and soups with you wherever you go!

www.kleankanteen.com
This is my favorite company, not only for their great stainless steel water bottles of various sizes, but for their many different types of food canisters, cups, tumblers, and kids' bottles and sippy cups. It is worth a look if want an alternative to toxin-containing plastic food containers.

www.mightynest.com/shop
MightyNest offers a fantastic collection of glass, stainless steel, and other healthy non-plastic food storage containers, lunch containers, bottles, cups, insulated jars, thermoses, and any other tote from a wide range of companies.

SUPPLEMENTS, POWDERS, AND OTHER EXTRAS

www.medicinenet.com/supplements -vitamins/article.htm
This site has a comprehensive list of nutrients and medicinal herbs, including their uses and warnings.

www.ods.od.nih.gov
The National Institutes of Health's Office of Dietary Supplements helps strengthen consumers' and wellness practitioners' knowledge and understanding of dietary supplements. Although it is conservative in bent, it is still a great place to poke around to learn more about nutrients.

www.vitacost.com
Vitacost carries an enormous range of supplements, herbs, protein powders, and other health items you may want for your detox.

SELF-CARE ITEMS

www.naturallivingideas.com
Natural Living Ideas is a great site filled with DIY ideas, articles on clean living, and more.

www.safecosmetics.org
The Campaign for Safe Cosmetics site has a wealth of information on the ingredients (both safe and questionable) in the self-care items we use on a daily basis. Because skin absorbs toxins, it's important to use clean cosmetics while you are detoxing. This site can help you do that!

www.wellnessmama.com
I have always enjoyed this site! Wellness Mama is a treasure trove of information on chemical-free living. It has fun articles, a great blog, and recipes for a wide range of self-care items.

CLEAN CLOTHING

www.bluecanoe.com
Blue canoe is a fashion-forward line of

US-made clothing made completely from cloth woven from organic hemp or organic cotton.

www.maggiesorganics.com
Maggie's Organics makes beautiful scarves, hats, and socks for babies, children, men, and women out of organic cotton. There are some gorgeous skirts, leggings, and tops.

www.synergyclothing.com
Synergy Clothing has stunning women's clothing made from organic fabrics. Synergy's high-fashion clothing is a bit pricier than what you'd find at a mainstream clothing store chain, but they are made in the United States and come in a range of sizes (from petite to plus), and a portion of the proceeds goes to good causes around the globe. These are clothes you can wear to the office, as well as for formal occasions.

CLEAN HOME
www.chemical-free-living.com
This site is an e-commerce site that also features articles on every aspect of clean living, including recipes and product recommendations.

www.eartheasy.com
A combination online store and blog, Earth Easy offers pre-made home products, as well as recipes and articles to help you get the chemicals out of your home.

www.nontoxic.com
This online store is a great resource for anyone aiming to create a nontoxic home with toxin-free carpeting, paint, tapestries, air filters, water purifiers, and more. It also includes articles and FAQs.

SPIRITUAL SUPPLIES
www.healyourlife.com
Created by the self-help guru Louise Hay, Heal Your Life features a smorgasbord of spiritual activities, from oracle cards to affirmations.

www.innerpath.com
When individuals detox, it is common for them to become more spiritual—or at least more interested in spirituality. Inner Path offers a range of products to help with meditation, yoga, feng shui, and other mindful pursuits.

BOOKS YOU MAY LIKE
Balanced Raw: Combine Raw and Cooked Foods for Optimal Health, Weight Loss, and Vitality Burst: A Four-Week Program, by Tina Leigh (Fair Winds Press). *Balanced Raw* is perfect for anyone flirting with going raw or who enjoys eating uncooked food but doesn't want to commit to an entirely raw lifestyle.

Clean Food, Revised Edition: A Seasonal Guide to Eating Close to the Source, by Terry Walters (Sterling Epicure). *Clean Food* is a feast for the senses that will nourish mind, body, and soul. Gluten-free eaters will find recipes throughout the book to meet their needs.

Coconut: The Complete Guide to the World's Most Versatile Superfood, by Stephanie Pedersen (Sterling). *Coconut* makes it easy to add this delicious healing food to your daily diet in many forms, including dried, fresh, water, milk, cream, butter, amino acids, sugar, and nectar.

Kale: The Complete Guide to the World's Most Powerful Superfood, by Stephanie

Pedersen (Sterling). The best-selling book on kale continues to show readers how to add kale to their breakfasts, lunches, dinners, desserts, and snacks. Getting your daily dose of this potent superfood is both easy and delicious.

Powerful Plant-Based Superfoods: The Best Way to Eat for Maximum Health, Energy, and Weight Loss, by Lauri Boone (Fair Winds Press). This book gives a wonderful rundown of superfoods, what they do, which to use for specific ailments, and how to enjoy them.

Wild About Greens: 125 Delectable Vegan Recipes for Kale, Collards, Arugula, Bok Choy, and Other Leafy Veggies Everyone Loves, by Nava Atlas (Sterling Epicure). Detoxifying cruciferous veggies, Asian greens, and many other leafy foods are a breeze to grow and prepare—and these 125 recipes showcase the most commonly used varieties in a wide selection of flavorful dishes.

WEBSITES YOU MAY LIKE

www.StephaniePedersen.com

This is the author's website, where you can learn more about detoxing, read health articles, explore recipes, and become part of Stephanie's online circle of friends.

www.HighImpactHealth.com

This is the author's training site, designed to help health coaches, nutritionists, and other wellness practitioners rock their businesses with training, certification programs, and marketing help.

www.eco-farm.org

The Ecological Farming Association nurtures healthy farms, food systems, and communities.

www.ewg.org

The Environmental Working Group's website helps individuals avoid environmental pollution in the air, in the food supply, and everywhere else. Check out the organization's famous "Dirty Dozen" and "Clean Fifteen" lists, which help shoppers decide where they can save money by purchasing mainstream produce, and where it is essential that they go organic.

www.foodandwaterwatch.org

This site offers a look at the politics and players in today's food industries.

www.nutrition.org

The American Society for Nutrition stands for excellence in nutrition research and science.

www.organicconsumers.org

The Organic Consumers Association helps maintain organic food standards.

www.panna.org

Pesticide Action Network provides information about harmful pesticides and works to replace pesticide use with ecologically sound and socially just alternatives.

www.centerforfoodsafety.org

The Center for Food Safety works to protect human health and the environment by curbing the proliferation of harmful food production technologies and by promoting organic and other forms of sustainable agriculture.

www.whfoods.com

The World's Healthiest Foods is the fabulously information-dense website for the George Mateljan Foundation, a not-for-profit foundation that helps individuals make more informed decisions about the foods they choose to eat.

METRIC EQUIVALENTS: LIQUID

This chart can also be used for small amounts of dry ingredients,
such as salt and baking powder.

U.S. quantity	Metric equivalent	U.S. quantity	Metric equivalent
¼ teaspoon	1 ml	⅛ cup	30 ml
½ teaspoon	2.5 ml	¼ cup (2 fluid ounces)	60 ml
¾ teaspoon	4 ml	⅓ cup	80 ml
1 teaspoon	5 ml	½ cup (4 fluid ounces)	120 ml
1¼ teaspoons	6 ml	⅔ cup	160 ml
1½ teaspoons	7.5 ml	¾ cup (6 fluid ounces)	180 ml
1¾ teaspoons	8.5 ml	1 cup (8 fluid ounces)	240 ml
2 teaspoons	10 ml	1½ cups (12 fluid ounces)	350 ml
1 tablespoon	15 ml	3 cups	700 ml
2 tablespoons	30 ml	4 cups (1 quart)	950 ml (.95 liter)

METRIC EQUIVALENTS: DRY

Ingredient	1 cup	¾ cup	⅔ cup	½ cup	⅓ cup	¼ cup	2 tbsp
All-purpose gluten-free flour	160g	120g	106g	80g	53g	40g	20g
Granulated sugar	200g	150g	130g	100g	65g	50g	25g
Confectioners' sugar	100g	75g	70g	50g	35g	25g	13g
Brown sugar, firmly packed	180g	135g	120g	90g	60g	45g	23g
Cornmeal	160g	120g	100g	80g	50g	40g	20g
Cornstarch	120g	90g	80g	60g	40g	30g	15g
Shortening	190g	140g	125g	95g	65g	48g	24g
Chopped fruits and vegetables	150g	110g	100g	75g	50g	40g	20g
Chopped seeds	150g	110g	100g	75g	50g	40g	20g
Ground seeds	120g	90g	80g	60g	40g	30g	15g

ACKNOWLEDGMENTS

I couldn't have finished *The 7-Day Superfood Cleanse* without the support of my husband, Richard Joseph Demler, and our sons, Leif Christian Pedersen, Anders Gyldenvalde Pedersen, and Axel SuneLund Pedersen. Thanks, too, to the NYC wellness community, which is a surprisingly tight-knit, happy group of healers who have reminded me to have fun as I have literally lived detoxing for several months!

Thanks to so many friends who supported my family and me during the book-writing process. Oceana, our morning check-ins are so powerful. They allow me to sit down to a day of writing with a sense of focus and fun. Lola, you incorrigible flirt, you. I must acknowledge your cheeky sense of fun, which never fails to surprise me (I adore happy surprises!) and make me laugh. Laughing is so energizing, don't you think? The perfect way to refresh the spirit and clear the head!

I want to give a shout-out to the Saint Thomas Choir School for taking such outstanding care of Leif and Anders as I wrote: headmaster, housemothers, choir director, organists, teachers, gap students, tutor, school chef, and all of you. Your just-watchful-enough eyes and encouragement perfectly supported my kids, freeing up the mental energy I needed to write. Thank you from the bottom of my heart. And thanks, too, to my choir school parent friends who have become family: You rock. Dina Erickson, your exquisite care and championing of Leif and Anders has made you their favorite mother of all time. I appreciate you and your hilarious hubby, Peter Erickson.

Thanks to my amazing detox clients for the constant inspiration you bring. I run a number of different group cleanses, including a 5-Day Cleanse, a 7-Day Cleanse, and a 21-Day Cleanse. Each time I run one of these detox programs, I get the chance to be amazed at your drive, your courage, your curiosity, and your will. Cleansing can seem a bit scary, and yet you understand the joy in feeling your best, dive in, and create vibrant wellness for yourselves. Yay, you! I am in awe of each of you!

I can't say enough flattering (and true!) things about my gorgeous, good-humored, brilliant editor, Jennifer Williams. We go back in time through several publishing houses now. I count my blessings that I was assigned, as a young author, to you all those years ago. Here's to us! My designer, Christine Heun, ensured that this book is as polished and professional-looking as it is! Bill Milne created the gorgeous, mouthwatering photos in *The 7-Day Superfood Cleanse*. And my very thorough production editor, Kim Broderick, kept us all on schedule, while seeing to all the details with her usual equanimity and patience. Thank you! Your calm, can-do demeanor and overall smarty-pants ways make this crazy business of publishing look glamorous.

Thanks so much to my publicity pro, Sherri McLendon, of Professional Moneta. Sherri, I adore our monthly conversations. Not only are you fun and witty (and you know how much I love witty people), you make my professional life so much easier, which in turn makes my professional life more fun!

Lastly, I must thank you, dear reader, for your interest. Thank you!

Stephanie

INDEX

A

Acidity and alkalinity, 48–49, 168
Acne, mask for, 137
Alcohol, cleanses and, 37, 122, 166
Alkalinity, pH and, 48–49, 168
Aluminum, toxicity of, 79
Animal foods, reducing/
  eliminating, 15–18, 165–166
Anthocyanins, 85
Apple cider vinegar, benefits of, 13
Avocado
  about: benefits and uses, 3
  Avocado-Coconut Dip, 113
  Avocado Coconut Mask, 138
  Chopped Avocado Coconut
    Salad, 124

B

Baked Kale Chips, 107
Bananas
  Anti-Acne Mask, 137
  Banana Pre-Conditioner, 134
Bathing tips/products. *See*
  Self-care
Beach Body Polish Recipe, 142
Beans and other legumes
  about: making ahead, 162;
    shopping list, 26–27
  Black-Eyed Pea Salad, 83
  Braised Coconut Spinach
    and Chickpeas with
    Lemon, 93
  Dinner Salad Blueprint, 123
  Dinner Soup Blueprint, 117
  Grain or Bean Salad
    Blueprint, 80
  Hummus, 111
  Mexicali Quinoa Pilaf, 84
  Quinoa Superfood Salad, 81
  Roasted Coconut Chickpeas,
    106
  White Bean Dip, 112
Bedtime snacks, 38, 128
Beets
  about: kidney stones and, 46
  Celeriac and Beet Salad, 125
  Roasted Veggies in Coconut
    Oil, 94

Superfood Beet Soup, 119
Winter Pink Drink: Blender
  Version, 59
Winter Pink Drink: Juicer
  Version, 60
Black-Eyed Pea Salad, 83
Blender drinks
  about: blender brand
    recommendations, 51,
    55; blender safety and,
    52–53; blending green
    drinks on road, 55; need
    for blender, 169–170;
    sources for blenders, 171
  Carrot Lassi, 62
  Citrus Zinger, 62
  Coconut Cooler, 63
  Green Drink Blender
    Blueprint, 54–55, 70–71
  Key Lime–Coconut Frappé,
    64
  Summer Watermelon Detox
    Smoothie, 61
  Winter Pink Drink: Blender
    Version, 59
Bloating
  avoiding foods causing, iv, 24
  coffee and. *See* Coffee,
    eliminating
  coming off of cleanse and, 147,
    148, 154–155
  identifying cause of, 154
  rebooting cleanse for, 154–155
Body care. *See* Self-care
Books, other resources, 173–174
BPA (bisphenol A), toxicity
  of, 78
Braised Coconut Spinach and
  Chickpeas with Lemon, 93
Breakfast, 69–75
  about: additional food for, 73;
    coming off of cleanse, 149;
    green drinks for, 32–33,
    167–168; ideal for detox,
    69; meal plan (Everyday
    Cleanse Plan), 32–33;
    meal plan (Quick Release
    Plan), 39–40; not wanting

to eat, 162–163; overview
  of, 69; vegetables for, 163;
  weight loss and, 69
  alternatives to green drinks,
    74–75
  Green Drink Blender
    Blueprint, 70–71
  Green Drink Juicer Blueprint,
    72–73
Breast-feeding, cleanse and, 170
Breathing techniques, 43–44
Brightening Mask, 139
Broccoli rabe, sautéed, 97
Brown rice. *See* Rice
Brushing skin, 34
Bug repellent, homemade, 143
Burroughs, Stanley, 57

C

Caffeine, 6, 14, 30, 65, 103
Calories, equality of, 115
Carrots
  Carrot Lassi, 62
  Carrot Soup, 120
  Roasted Veggies in Coconut
    Oil, 94
  Winter Pink Drink: Blender
    Version, 59
  Winter Pink Drink: Juicer
    Version, 60
Celeriac and Beet Salad, 125
Chard. *See* Swiss chard
Chewing, importance of, 33
Chia
  about: benefits and uses, 3, 99;
    to buy, 27
  Chia Fresca, 100
  Chia Pudding, 101
Chickpeas. *See* Beans and other
  legumes
Chips. *See* Snacks
Chopped Avocado Coconut
  Salad, 124
Citrus
  about: "Lemonade Diet"
    Master Cleanse, 57
  Bath Fizzles, 141
  Brightening Mask, 139

Citrus Zinger, 62
Classic Lemon-Ginger Tea, 66
Green Drink Blender Blueprint, 54–55, 70–71
Green Drink Juicer Blueprint, 56–57, 72–73
Key Lime–Coconut Frappé, 64
Lemon Ginger Detox Drink, 64
Lemon Water, 63
Tahini Lemon Dressing, 130
Winter Pink Drink: Blender Version, 59
Winter Pink Drink: Juicer Version, 60
Classic Greens, 95
Classic Lemon-Ginger Tea, 66
Cleanses (detoxes). See also Preparing for cleanse; 7-Day Superfood Cleanse
alcohol and, 37, 122
benefits of, v–vi
duration of, iv–v
mindset for, 29–31
negative effects to avoid, 2
popularity of, iv–v
purpose of, vi
safety of, 156
short, advantages of, vii–viii
speeding up, vi
Clothing, resources for, 172–173
Clutter, clearing, 41
Cocktails, alcohol and, 37, 122, 166
Coconut
about: benefits and uses, 4; ingredients to buy, 26, 27
Avocado-Coconut Dip, 113
Braised Coconut Spinach and Chickpeas with Lemon, 93
Chopped Avocado Coconut Salad, 124
Coconut Brown Rice, 89
Coconut Chips Using a Mature Coconut, 105
Coconut Cooler, 63
Coconut Quinoa, 90
Key Lime–Coconut Frappé, 64

personal care products with. See Self-care
Roasted Coconut Chickpeas, 106
Spicy Pumpkin Coconut Bisque, 118
Coconut oil, 27
Coffee, eliminating, 12–15, 65, 165
Cold, feeling, 159
Collards, 26, 95
Colonics, 169
Constipation, 157
Containers, non-toxic, 87
Cooking concerns/solutions, 161, 162
Cosmetics. See Self-care
Cranberries
about: benefits and uses, 4
Winter Pink Drink: Blender Version, 59
Winter Pink Drink: Juicer Version, 60
Cravings
alcohol and, 166
apple cider vinegar and, 13
assessing detox need and, 6
causes of, iv, 14, 15, 74
coffee triggering, 14, 165
gluten and, 18, 166
handling/eliminating, iv, v, 3, 32, 48, 76, 103, 163, 167–168
sleep, fatigue and, 30
sugar, 20, 30, 165
Crudités, 103
Cucumbers
about: shopping list, 26
Green Drink Blender Blueprint, 54–55, 70–71
Green Drink Juicer Blueprint, 56–57, 72–73
Summer Watermelon Detox Smoothie, 61

D
Dairy, reducing/eliminating, 15–18, 166
Dairy, weight loss and, 16–17
Desk, eating at, 88–89
Detoxes. See Cleanses (detoxes); 7-Day Superfood Cleanse

Digestion concerns, 156–159
Dining out, 24–25, 77
Dinner, 115–131. See also Salad dressings; Soups about: coming off of cleanse, 150; evening cocktails and, 122; meal plan (Everyday Cleanse Plan), 37–38; meal plan (Quick Cleanse Plan), 42–44; overview of, 115–116; salads for, 122
Celeriac and Beet Salad, 125
Chopped Avocado Coconut Salad, 124
Dinner Salad Blueprint, 123
Nutty Kale Salad, 126
Dips
about, 110
Avocado-Coconut Dip, 113
Easy Pumpkin Protein Dip, 113
Garlicky Kale and Spinach Dip, 114
Hummus, 111
Raw Zucchini Hummus, 110
White Bean Dip, 112
Drinks, 59–69. See also Green Drink Blueprints; Green drinks
about: detox teas, 65–66; importance of, 45–46; overview of, 59; teas to buy/stock, 27
Carrot Lassi, 62
Chia Fresca, 100
Citrus Zinger, 62
Classic Lemon-Ginger Tea, 66
Coconut Cooler, 63
Key Lime–Coconut Frappé, 64
Lemon Ginger Detox Drink, 64
Lemon Water, 63
Stomach Soother, 67
Summer Watermelon Detox Smoothie, 61
Turmeric Tea, 68
Winter Pink Drink: Blender Version, 59
Winter Pink Drink: Juicer Version, 60

E

Easy Pumpkin Protein Dip, 113
Eating issues, 162–163
Eggs, not eating, 15, 165
Emotional eating disorders, 170
Enzymes, importance of, 71
Evening, relaxing in, 127
Everyday Cleanse Plan. *See* Meal plans: Everyday Cleanse Plan
Evolution Juice, 74–75
Exfoliating skin, 34
Extending cleanse, 152–153
Extreme Pop-Up Mini-Cleanse, 155
Eye cream, coconut, 146

F

FAQs, 164–170
Fatigue, 159
Food. *See also* specific main ingredients
    chewing sufficiently, 33
    choices, for cleanse, 23–25
    eating concerns, 162–163
    eating out, 24–25, 77
    flexibility with, 25
    importance of, 23
    optional, 28
    reducing/eliminating animal foods, 15–18
    reducing/eliminating gluten, 18, 166
    reducing/eliminating soy, 19
    reducing sugar intake, 19–20
    restricted, list and rationale, 24
    special diets and, 31, 45
    to stock/shopping list, 25–28
    water-retaining, avoiding, 24
Fruit, cleanse and, 49, 74, 167
Fullness, feeling of, 158–159

G

Garlicky Kale and Spinach Dip, 114
Ginger
    Classic Lemon-Ginger Tea, 66
    Gingered Millet with Japanese Veggies, 82–83
    Ginger-Sunflower Seed Dressing, 131
    Lemon Ginger Detox Drink, 64
Gluten, reducing/eliminating, 18, 166
Goals, setting, 10–11
Grains. *See also* Millet; Rice
    about: shopping list for, 27; veggies with, 86, 91
    Grain or Bean Salad Blueprint, 80
Green Drink Blueprints
    about: blender recommendations, 51, 55; blender safety tips, 52–53; making when traveling, 55; overview of, 51–52; thyroid disorders and, 58; using after cleanse, 52
    Green Drink Blender Blueprint, 54–55, 70–71
    Green Drink Juicer Blueprint, 56–57, 72–73
Green drinks
    alternative juice options, 74–75, 162
    benefits of, 43
    best time to drink, 21
    blending on road, 55
    bottled, 74–75
    breakfast meal plan, 32–33
    as cornerstone of cleanse, 47
    enzyme importance and, 71
    experimenting with, 21–22
    importance of, 21, 43, 45–49
    kidney stones and, 46
    learning to enjoy, 21–22
    in morning, 32–33, 167–168. *See also* Breakfast
    overview of, 46–47
    pH levels and, 48–49
    protein and, 33, 67
    safety precaution, 45
    shopping list for, 26
    special diets and, 45
    thyroid disorders and, 58
    tips for making appetizing, 49–51
Greens. *See also* Kale; Salads; Spinach

Classic Greens, 95
Indian Greens, 96

H

Hair-care products. *See* Self-care
Hardcore option. *See* Meal plans: Quick Cleanse Plan
Headaches, 158
Herbs, to buy, 26
Home, clean, 173
Hummus recipes, 110, 111
Hunger, 158

I

Indian Greens, 96
Ingredients. *See also* specific main ingredients
    optional, 28
    to stock/shopping list, 25–28
    unappealing, 25
Irritability, 158

J

Juicing and juices
    about: commercial juices as green drink alternatives, 74–75; fresh-pressed from store, 75; need for juicer, 169–170; sources for juicers, 171; using watermelon rinds, 61
    Green Drink Juicer Blueprint, 56–57, 72–73
    Winter Pink Drink: Juicer Version, 60

K

Kale
    about: benefits and uses, 4; shopping list, 26
    Baked Kale Chips, 107
    Classic Greens, 95
    Garlicky Kale and Spinach Dip, 114
    Nutty Kale Salad, 126
    Salt and Vinegar Kale Chips, 108
Key Lime–Coconut Frappé, 64
Kidney stones, 46, 48, 168
Kitchen, health-supportive, 20–21, 24. *See also* Food

L

Lead, toxicity of, 79
Lemon and lime. *See* Citrus
Lettuce. *See* Green Drink
   Blueprints; Salads
Lifestyle concerns, 159–161
Lunch, 76–97
   about: coming off of cleanse,
      149–150; complete meal
      options, 77–78; eating at
      desk (precautions), 88–89;
      grains with veggies, 86, 91;
      habits to avoid, 88–89; ideal
      for detox, 76; meal plan
      (Everyday Cleanse Plan),
      36–37; meal plan (Quick
      Cleanse Plan), 40–42; non-
      toxic ways to pack, 87;
      overview of, 76; takeout
      options, 77, 78–79, 162;
      toxins to avoid, 78–79
   Black-Eyed Pea Salad, 83
   Black Rice Salad, 85
   Braised Coconut Spinach
      and Chickpeas with
      Lemon, 93
   Brown Rice Medley, 86
   Classic Greens, 95
   Coconut Brown Rice, 89
   Coconut Quinoa, 90
   Gingered Millet with Japanese
      Veggies, 82–83
   Grain or Bean Salad Blueprint,
      80
   Indian Greens, 96
   Mexicali Quinoa Pilaf, 84
   Millet with Roasted Sunflower
      Seeds, 87
   Quinoa Superfood Salad, 81
   Roasted Veggies in Coconut
      Oil, 94
   Sautéed Broccoli Rabe, 97
   Side Salad Blueprint, 92

M

Maple Dijon Vinaigrette, 130
Masks. *See* Self-care
Master Cleanse ("Lemonade
   Diet"), 57
Meal plans
   about: overview of, 31
   days 1–7. *See* Meal plans:

Everyday Cleanse Plan
   enhanced. *See* Meal plans:
   Quick Cleanse Plan
   menu options, 164–165
Meal plans: Everyday Cleanse
   Plan, 32–38
   about, 31; Quick Cleanse Plan
      and, 31; special diets and,
      31, 45
   breakfast, 32–33
   coming off of cleanse, 147–151
   dinner, 37–38
   extending cleanse, 152–153
   lunch, 36–37
   snacks, 35–36, 38, 128
   throughout day, 32
Meal plans: Quick Cleanse Plan
   about: breakfast meal plan,
      39–40; as optional hard
      core option, 39; overview
      of, 9, 31, 39
   breakfast, 39–40
   before breakfast/upon waking,
      39
   coming off of cleanse, 147–151
   dinner, 42–44
   extending cleanse, 152–153
   lunch, 40–42
   snacks, 40, 42, 43, 128
   throughout day, 39
Meat, reducing/eliminating,
   15–18, 166
Metric equivalents, 175
Mexicali Quinoa Pilaf, 84
Millet
   about: making ahead, 162;
      shopping list, 27
   Gingered Millet with Japanese
      Veggies, 82–83
   Millet with Roasted Sunflower
      Seeds, 87
Mindset, for cleanse, 29–31
Mini-cleanse, 155
Mint, in Stomach Soother, 67
Moisturizers. *See* Self-care

N

Night, avoiding eating at, 169.
   See also Bedtime snacks
Nuts and seeds. *See also* Chia
   about: butters, 27; pepitas
      benefits and uses, 4–5;

shopping list, 27; walnuts
   benefits and uses, 5
Creamy Salad Dressing
   Blueprint, 129
Ginger-Sunflower Seed
   Dressing, 131
Millet with Roasted Sunflower
   Seeds, 87
Nutty Kale Salad, 126
Stomach Soother, 67
Tahini Lemon Dressing, 130

O

Office, eating at, 88–89, 169
Olive oil, 27

P

Pepitas. *See* Nuts and seeds
Personal care. *See* Self-care
pH levels, 48–49, 168
Phthalates, toxicity of, 79
Pomegranate
   about: benefits and uses, 5
   Quinoa Superfood Salad, 81
Pop-up cleanses, 154–155
Potatoes, in Roasted Veggies in
   Coconut Oil, 94
Pregnancy, cleanse and, 170
Preparing for cleanse
   about: overview of, 12
   apple cider vinegar and, 13
   eliminating coffee, 12–15, 65
   goal setting, 10–11
   importance of, 23
   increasing water intake, 12,
      32, 168
   kitchen preparation, 20–21, 24
   mindset preparation, 29–31
   reducing/eliminating animal
      foods, 15–18, 165–166
   reducing/eliminating gluten,
      18, 166
   reducing/eliminating soy, 19
   reducing sugar intake, 19–20,
      165
   scheduling considerations,
      22, 29
   shopping list, 25–28
   sleep schedule and, 30
   telling others about, 29–30
   trying green drink, 21–22.
      See also Green Drink
      Blueprints

Press Juice juices, 75
Processed foods, 167
Protein, green drinks and, 33, 67
Pudding, chia, 101
Pumpkin
  about: pepitas benefits and
    uses, 4–5
  Easy Pumpkin Protein Dip, 113
  Spicy Pumpkin Coconut
    Bisque, 118
PVC (polyvinyl chloride), toxicity
  of, 78–79

Q

Quick Cleanse Plan. *See* Meal
  plans: Quick Cleanse Plan
Quinoa
  about: benefits and uses, 5;
    making ahead, 162;
    shopping list, 27
  Coconut Quinoa, 90
  Mexicali Quinoa Pilaf, 84
  Quinoa Superfood Salad, 81

R

Raw Zucchini Hummus, 110
Rebooting cleanse, 154–155
Relaxing in evening, 127
Resources, 171–174
Restaurant, eating at, 24–25, 77
Rice
  about: making ahead, 162;
    shopping list, 27
  Black Rice Salad, 85
  Brown Rice Medley, 86
  Coconut Brown Rice, 89
  Roasted Coconut Chickpeas,
    106

S

Salad dressings, 128–131
  about: overview of, 128
  Creamy Salad Dressing
    Blueprint, 129
  Ginger-Sunflower Seed
    Dressing, 131
  Maple Dijon Vinaigrette,
    130
  Tahini Lemon Dressing, 130
Salads
  about: for breakfast, 74; for
    dinner, 122; in place of

green drink, 74; shopping
    list for, 26
  Black-Eyed Pea Salad, 83
  Celeriac and Beet Salad, 125
  Chopped Avocado Coconut
    Salad, 124
  Dinner Salad Blueprint, 123
  Grain or Bean Salad
    Blueprint, 80
  Nutty Kale Salad, 126
  Side Salad Blueprint, 92
Salt and Vinegar Kale Chips, 108
Salt Detox Bath Recipe, 133
Sautéed Broccoli Rabe, 97
Scheduling detoxes, 22, 29
Seeds. *See* Chia; Nuts and seeds
Self-care, 132–146
  about: better-for-you cosmetics,
    132; facial products, 137;
    hair-care products, 133–
    134; hand and body care,
    140; overview of detoxing
    and, 132; product resources,
    172; for teeth and eyes, 145
  Anti-Acne Mask, 137
  Avocado Coconut Mask, 138
  Banana Pre-Conditioner, 134
  Bath Fizzles, 141
  Beach Body Polish Recipe,
    142
  Brightening Mask, 139
  Coconut Detangler, 136
  Coconut Eye Cream, 146
  Homemade Bug Repellent,
    143
  Homemade Sugar Scrub, 143
  Homemade Sunscreen, 144
  Homemade Toothpaste with
    Coconut Oil, 145
  Nourishing Body wash, 140
  Salt Detox Bath Recipe, 133
  Semi-Homemade Shampoo,
    136
  Totally Coconut Pre-Shampoo
    Hair Mask, 135
  Whipped Body Butter, 143
  Whipped Coconut
    Moisturizer, 139
Senses, heightening of, 157
7-Day Superfood Cleanse. *See
  also* Superfoods
  about: overview of, 7–8

alcohol and, 37, 122, 166
apple cider vinegar and, 13
assessing appropriateness for
    you, 6–7
benefits of, v–vi
breathing techniques, 43–44
chewing food and, 33
cleanse popularity and, iv–v
clearing clutter and, 41
coming off of, 147–151
compared to other cleanses,
    1–2
contraindications for, 170
eating out during, 24–25, 77
Everyday Cleanse Plan. *See*
    Meal plans: Everyday
    Cleanse Plan
exfoliating skin and, 34
extending, 152–153
FAQs, 164–170
food choices for, 23–25
mindset for, 29–31
pop-up cleanses, 154–155
preparing for. *See* Preparing
    for cleanse
questions to ask before, 6–7
Quick Cleanse Plan. *See* Meal
    plans: Quick Cleanse Plan
rebooting, 154–155
relaxing in evening, 127
safety of, 156
short-cleanse advantages,
    vii–viii
sleep and, 30
special diets and, 31, 45
sweating and, 24
telling others about, 29–30
uniqueness of, vi–vii
Shampoo. *See* Self-care
Sharing cleanse information,
    29–30
Shopping
  budget concerns, 161
  bulk food sources, 171
  list, 25–28
Side Salad Blueprint, 92
Skin, brushing, 34
Skincare. *See* Self-care
Sleep, 30
Snacks. *See also* Dips
  about: author's favorites, 109;
    before bed, 38, 128;

coming off of cleanse, 149, 150, 151; creamy treats, 99; defined, 104; Everyday Cleanse Plan, 35; overview of snacking and, 98; Quick Release Plan, 40, 42–43; statistics on, 102; veggies as, 102
Baked Kale Chips, 107
Chia Fresca, 100
Chia Pudding, 101
Coconut Chips Using a Mature Coconut, 105
Crudités, 103
Roasted Coconut Chickpeas, 106
Salt and Vinegar Kale Chips, 108
Soups
about: to buy, 26; making ahead, 162; overview of, 116
Carrot Soup, 120
Dinner Soup Blueprint, 117
Simple Tomato Soup, 121
Spicy Pumpkin Coconut Bisque, 118
Superfood Beet Soup, 119
Soy, reducing/eliminating, 19
Spicy Pumpkin Coconut Bisque, 118
Spinach
about: kidney stones and, 46; shopping list, 26
Braised Coconut Spinach and Chickpeas with Lemon, 93
Garlicky Kale and Spinach Dip, 114
Green Drink Blender Blueprint, 54–55, 70–71
Green Drink Juicer Blueprint, 56–57, 72–73
Spiritual supplies, 173
Squash. See also Pumpkin
Brown Rice Medley, 86
Mexicali Quinoa Pilaf, 84
Raw Zucchini Hummus, 116
Roasted Veggies in Coconut Oil, 94
Stomach Soother, 67

Storage supplies, 172
Sugar intake, 19–20, 165
Sugar scrub, 143
Suja green drinks, 75
Summer Watermelon Detox Smoothie, 61
Sunscreen, homemade, 144
Superfood Beet Soup, 119
Superfoods
about: 7-Day Superfood Cleanse and, vii
benefits/power of, 2–5, 23
other names for, 2, 23
shopping list, 25–28
types and benefits, 3–5
weight loss, health and, 2
Supplement, resources for, 172
Sweating, value of, 24
Sweet potatoes, in Roasted Veggies in Coconut Oil, 94
Swiss chard
about: greens shopping list, 26; kidney stones and, 46
Indian Greens, 96

T
Tahini Lemon Dressing, 130
Takeout lunches, 77, 78–79, 162
Tea, detox, 65–66. See also Drinks
Thyroid disorders, green drinks and, 58
Timing, of detox, 22, 29
Tomato soup, 121
Toothpaste, homemade, 145
Toxins
avoiding in lunchbox, 78–79
non-toxic ways to pack lunch, 87
Travel, blending green drinks on road, 55
Troubleshooting, 156–163
eating concerns, 162–163
health/digestion concerns, 156–159
lifestyle concerns, 159–161
shopping, cooking, meal prep, 161–162
Turmeric Tea, 68

V
Vegetables. See also Salads; specific vegetables
about: for breakfast, 163; bulk sources, 171; chiffonade cutting technique, 126; grains with, 86, 91; safe for thyroid disorders, 58; shopping list, 26, 27–28; superfood, 27–28. See also Superfoods
Crudités, 103
Gingered Millet with Japanese Veggies, 82–83
Roasted Veggies in Coconut Oil, 94
Vinaigrette, maple Dijon, 130

W
Walnuts. See Nuts and seeds
Water intake, 12, 32, 168
Water, lemon, 63
Watermelon
about: using rinds in juice, 61
Summer Watermelon Detox Smoothie, 61
Water-retaining foods, avoiding, 24
Websites, resource, 174
Weight loss
apple cider vinegar and, 13
breakfast importance, 69
dairy and, 16–17
eating at night and, 169
mindful eating and, 88
troubleshooting, 158
White Bean Dip, 112
Winter Pink Drink: Blender Version, 59
Winter Pink Drink: Juicer Version, 60
Work, eating at, 88–89

Z
Zone, getting into. See Preparing for cleanse
Zucchini. See Squash

ABOUT THE AUTHOR

STEPHANIE PEDERSEN, MS, CHHC, is a holistic nutritionist, food educator, cookbook author, corporate speaker, and media host. Author of more than twenty books, Stephanie has a reputation for teaching people how to make nutrition easy, practical, and fun. She does this by using superfoods and other "power foods" to help individuals detoxify naturally, manage food allergies, eliminate cravings, and lose weight, using food and lifestyle changes.

As Stephanie says, "I want health for everyone. I have seen firsthand with myself and my own clients that when one works to get clean and fit and address one's health challenges, life gets bigger. Suddenly, life becomes outrageously fun and easy. You move healthfully through life with ease."

According to Stephanie, getting healthy doesn't have to be complicated or time-consuming. "As a mother, writer, nutritionist, educator and someone who loves to have time alone to wander local farmers markets, I know that complicated, overly fussy diets and an unnatural obsession with calorie-counting are not the answers to getting and staying healthy." Instead, Stephanie espouses a life of love, laughter, daily exercise, and your favorite whole foods. (Including plenty of superfoods!)

"We're lucky that we live in a time when more and more gorgeous whole food ingredients, organic produce, and humanely farmed meats are available. Let's celebrate our good fortune by exploring our many food and fitness options and experimenting with abandon."

Pedersen currently lives in New York City with her husband and three sons. Visit her at www.StephaniePedersen.com

Also by Stephanie Pedersen:

Coconut: The Complete Guide to the Most Versatile Superfood
Kale: The Complete Guide to the World's Most Powerful Superfood
The Pumpkin Pie Spice Cookbook
KISS Guide to Beauty: Keep It Simple Series
Shoes: What Every Woman Should Know
Bra: A Thousand Years of Style, Support, and Seduction

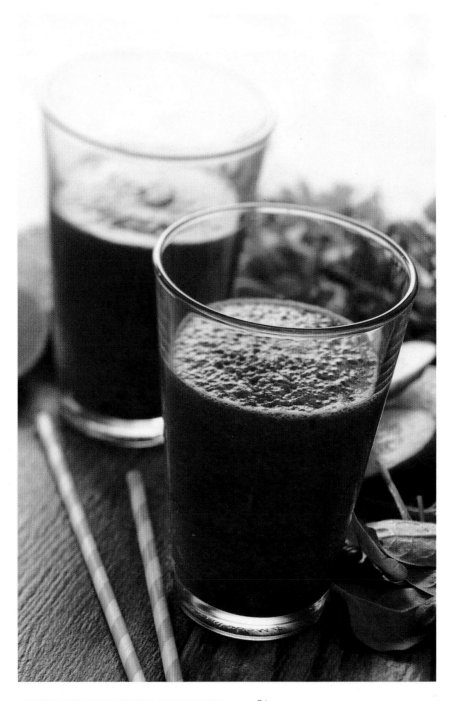

GREEN DRINK BLENDER BLUEPRINT, page 54

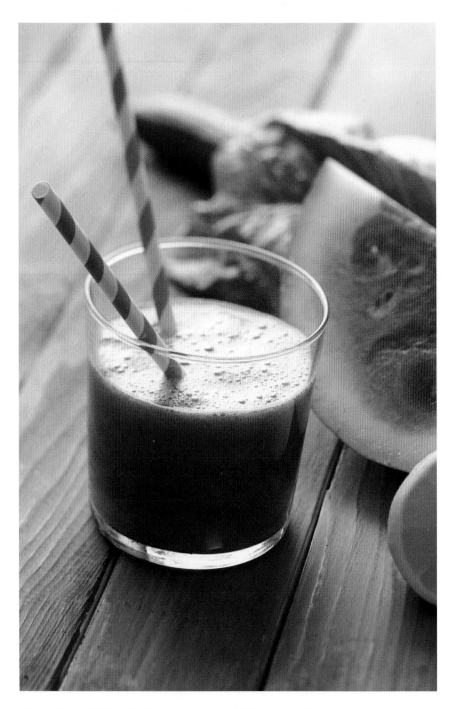

SUMMER WATERMELON DETOX SMOOTHIE, page 61

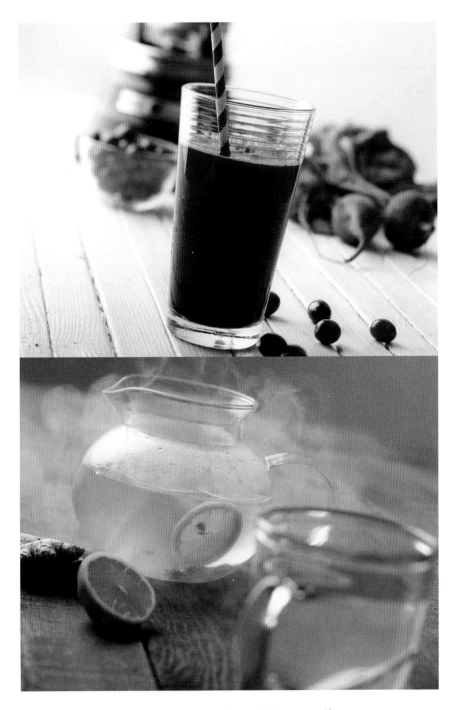

ABOVE: WINTER PINK DRINK: JUICER VERSION, page 60
BELOW: CLASSSIC LEMON-GINGER TEA, page 66

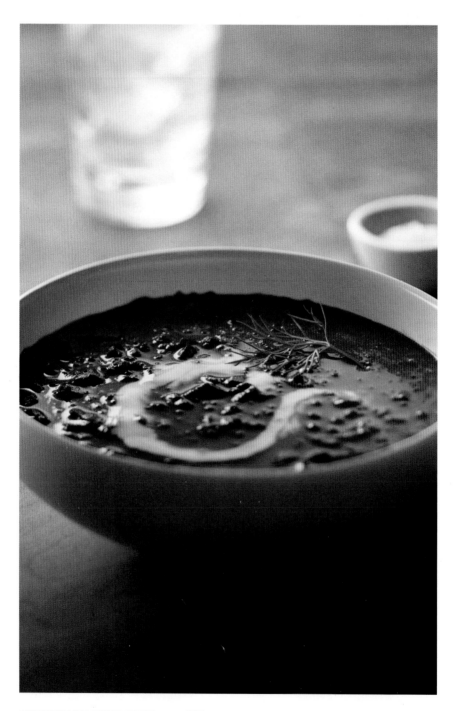

SUPERFOOD BEET SOUP, page 119

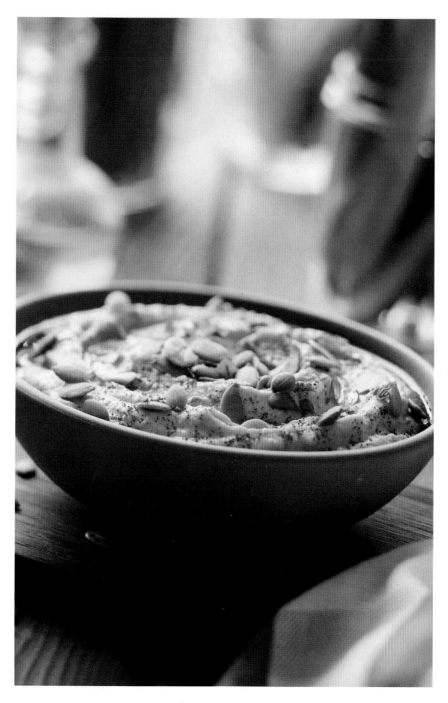

HUMMUS (garnished with pepitas, paprika, and herbs), page 111

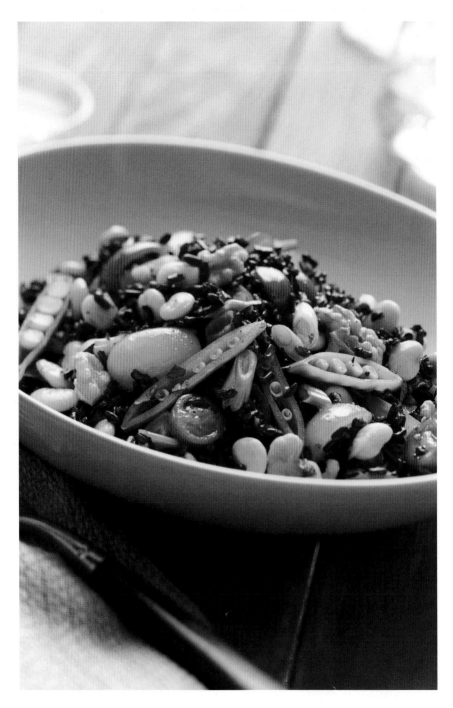

BLACK RICE SALAD, page 85